AGE-RELATED MACULAR DEGENERATION - ETIOLOGY, DIAGNOSIS AND MANAGEMENT - A GLANCE AT THE FUTURE

Edited by **Giuseppe Lo Giudice**

Age-Related Macular Degeneration - Etiology, Diagnosis and Management - A Glance at the Future
http://dx.doi.org/10.5772/56745
Edited by Giuseppe Lo Giudice

Contributors

KSimona Talu, Shani Golan, Anat Lowenstein, Jane Khan, Petr Kolar, Maria E Marin-Castano

Published by InTech

Janeza Trdine 9, 51000 Rijeka, Croatia

Notice

Publishing Process Manager Iva Simcic
Technical Editor InTech DTP team
Cover InTech Design team

Additional hard copies can be obtained from orders@intechopen.com

Age-Related Macular Degeneration - Etiology, Diagnosis and Management - A Glance at the Future,
Edited by Giuseppe Lo Giudice
p. cm.
ISBN 978-953-51-1113-9

For EU product safety concerns:
IN TECH d.o.o., Prolaz Marije Krucifikse Kozulić 3, 51000 Rijeka, Croatia,
info@intechopen.com or visit our website at intechopen.com.

Meet the editor

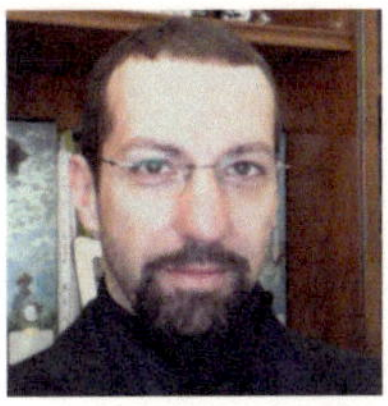

Dr. Lo Giudice is an Assistant professor of Ophthalmology at San Antonio Hospital in Padua (Italy),since 2007. He has more than 15 years of research experience in Age-related Macular Degeneration (AMD), in clinical trials and laboratory research, including genetic therapy for AMD, and development of new diagnostic tools for retinal degenerative disease. He collaborates with ophthalmologists and has authored or co-authored more than 40 papers in peer-reviewed journals. Dr. Lo Giudice received a MD from University of Messina (Italy) and MD in Ophthalmology from University of Padua in Italy.

Contents

Preface

Management of the patient affected by age-related macular degeneration (AMD) represents a paradigm challenge. Research has yielded major discoveries about the etiology, pathophysiology, and treatment of AMD over the last decade, although more steps are needed to continue to improve our know-how. The purpose of *"Age-related Macular Degeneration - Etiology, Diagnosis and Management - A Glance at the Future"* is to provide up-to-date information of the pathophysiology, diagnosis, management, and treatment of age-related macular degeneration. In this volume I have attempted to collect a significant amount of new information from retinal experts to first summarize the established information and then to present the most novel developments in their respective fields. The first section of this book includes the pathophysiology and epidemiology, of age-related macular degeneration. Oxidative damage to the RPE, extracellular matrix turnover, inflammation, and angiogenesis appear to be key cellular processes that play a central role in the pathogenesis of AMD. Some chapters will focus on the pathobiology of early stage AMD and its evolution to the later form also exploring the role of injury at the RPE in the onset and development of the disease. The second section focuses on the clinical features and diagnosis of age-related macular degeneration. The clinical findings seen in the nonexudative and exudative forms are discussed. The section on imaging includes a chapter on new OCT technology including: Swept Source OCT (SS-OCT), Enhanced Depth Imaging OCT (EDI-OCT), and adaptive optics. A variety of emerging OCT technologies are poised to expand significantly the scope of OCT imaging and to enhance significantly our approach to the diagnosis and management of patients with retinal disease. An in-depth understanding of these technologies and their potential advantages and disadvantages will aid retinal specialists in utilizing these new methods optimally. The next and last section reports information on current and experimental forms of treatment for non-exudative and exudative forms of age-related macular degeneration.

The advent of intravitreal anti-VEGF therapy (targeting all isoforms) dramatically altered the standard of care and treatment paradigms for patients with NVAMD. However, In spite of this significant step forward in the treatment of NVAMD, significant challenges remain. The presentation of the treatment options includes a discussion of the mechanism of action, the clinical treatment technique, the targeted patient population, as well as the expected outcomes of each treatment. No single manageable volume can analyze all of the existing knowledge concerning a disease such as age-related macular degeneration. Special attention has been paid to making the text easily readable. My sincere hope is that readers will find as much pleasure reading this textbook as I have had writing and editing it.

Dr. Giuseppe Lo Giudice
San Paolo Ophthalimc Center, San Antonio Hospital, Italy

To my father

Section 1

Epidemiology and Risk Factors

Chapter 1

AMD: Epidemiology and Risk Factors

Jane Khan

Additional information is available at the end of the chapter

http://dx.doi.org/10.5772/55234

1. Introduction

Age-related maculopathy (ARM) and age-related macular degeneration (AMD) are stages in a process of degeneration of the central macular region of the retina defined as occurring over the age of 50. This chapter examines the evidence for environmental and genetic risk factors for developing AMD.

2. Epidemiology

2.1. Burden and impact of disease

2.1.1. Incidence

Incidence rates for all ARM lesions increases significantly with age. In the Blue Mountains Eye Study (BMES) Mitchell et al found overall 5-year incidence of late ARM lesions (combined geographic atrophy and neovascular ARM), was 1.1%. Age specific rates were 0.0%, 0.6%, 2.4%, and 5.4% for participants aged 60 years and younger, 60 to 69 years, 70 to 79 years, and 80 years and older at baseline, respectively [1]. After excluding participants with either early or late ARM in either eye at baseline, the overall 5-year incidence of early ARM was 8.7%, (3.2%, 7.4%, 18.3%, and 14.8% for the corresponding age. The findings parallel those in the Beaver Dam Eye Study (BDES) where it was noted those 75 years of age or older have significantly higher 5-year incidence of exudative macular degeneration (1.8% vs. 0%), and pure geographic atrophy (1.7% vs. 0%) than people 43 to 54 years of age [2].

Individual ARM fundus signs that predict best the development of AMD are large drusen (> or =125 microm) [3], 10% or more of the grid area covered by drusen [3], soft indistinct drusen [2] and focal hyperpigmentation [2;4]. There is a high risk of second eye involvement with annual incidence of CNV occurring in the second eye of patients with CNV in the first eye reported as between 6-15% [5;6].

2.1.2. Prevalence

Age-related macular degeneration is the third largest world cause of visual impairment, and in Western countries it is often the leading cause of blindness. In the UK and USA for example it is the leading cause of blind registration [7;8 9;10] accounting for nearly 50% of blind and partial sight registrations in all age groups and nearly 55% in the over 65 age group. There is evidence to suggest the incidence of AMD is increasing. Evans and Wormald examined data from the Office of Population censuses and Surveys in the UK and compared available data for the years 1950, 1960, 1970 1980 and 1990 [11] and were able to demonstrate an increase in percentage registrations due to AMD by 30%. Population studies give prevalence figures of 2-10% for ARM in the age range 50-75. Thereafter, the frequency rapidly increases to figures of around 15% and nearing 50% in those over the age of 85. These prevalence figures vary according to the diagnostic criteria used hence the studies performed to date, with the exception of those using the International or Wisconsin grading systems, are difficult to compare. Whether or not the incidence is increasing there is no doubt that with the ageing population, the prevalence is increasing and the impact on the individual to be able to live independently will also have an indisputable impact on society.

2.2. Impact of AMD on the individual

2.2.1. Mortality

There is some evidence to suggest that poor vision is associated with increased mortality and co-morbidity in elderly people [12;13]; although interestingly those with much more severe visual impairment may actually live longer, perhaps due to leading more 'sheltered lives' [14]. However recent data suggest that AMD in itself is not associated with increased mortality but acts as a marker for other diseases which do [15].

2.2.2. Mental health, quality of life and well-being

Visual impairment has been shown to be more age-related than any other disability [7] and visually impaired elders may be at more risk of affective disorders, particularly depression [16]. Williams et al assessed the impact of AMD on quality of life and well-being [17]. The authors found significantly poorer ratings for quality of life and emotional distress in patients with AMD compared with age-matched adults and the rates were comparable with those reported for chronic illnesses (e.g. arthritis, bone marrow transplantees, chronic obstructive airways disease) [18]. Unpublished data (Jan Mitchell BSc, Royal Holloway, University of London) indicates that the Macular Disease Society Quality of Life questionnaire, incorporating the 12-item Well-being questionnaire [19], in addition to questions specifically designed to measure the impact of macular disease, showed a greater negative impact on most aspects of quality of life in macular degeneration compared with diabetes. In addition, attitudes of physicians was shown to add to the stress such a diagnosis may have on an individual by giving an impression of lack of concern or interest in their patients and by inadequate dissemination of information about the condition or services available to aid their rehabilitation [18]. In a study by Lee et al, blurred vision caused greater decrement in functioning and well-being than many other medical conditions including heart disease, diabetes, hypertension, indigestion and headaches. Only shortness of breath had a greater impact on these parameters than blurred vision [20]. The quality of life of community-dwelling elderly people has been shown to be significantly linked to sensory impairment. Mood level and social relationships are particularly affected by visual impairment [21]. A survey, using the VCM1 questionnaire [22] (a questionnaire designed to measure vision-related quality of life) lead to an estimate of more than 550,000 individuals in England with substantial vision-related quality of life impairment [23].

2.2.3. Falls and functional ability

Falls among the elderly are a major cause and result of morbidity and studies indicate that 30% of persons over the age of 65 may suffer a fall each year, increasing to 40% in those over 80 [24]. Tinetti et al demonstrated that although visual impairment was not the single most common cause of falls in the elderly it had a significant additive effect in this multifactorial condition [25]. Other studies have been able to show a significant positive association between reduced contrast sensitivity, reduced visual acuity and self-reported visual impairment [26;27] and falls. Older people tend to need to rely more on vision to maintain vertical posture [28]. Hip-fracture is clearly a serious consequence of falls in the elderly and has provided an objective outcome measure in assessing the relationship between poor vision and falls in the elderly. Cummings et al performed a detailed prospective study of 9516 white women over 65 years of age and found that poor contrast sensitivity and reduced depth perception were independent risk factors for hip fracture [29]. The Blue Mountains Eye Study has subsequently confirmed that measured visual impairment is associated with both falls and hip-fracture [30].

2.2.4. Driving and independence

Independence is an important measure of quality of life for older people. Being able to continue driving is often seen as the most valuable means of maintaining this independence. Macular degeneration and macular haemorrhage were found in one study to be among the six most frequent medical conditions for driving cessation in community-based ambulatory individuals over the age of 70 [31]. Evidence exists to show that older drivers with visual impairment and/or a constriction in the size of the useful field of view to be at greater risk for vehicle crashes than those without these problems [32]. Studies have also been able to show in more general terms loss of independence for example, in a survey by Branch et al of self-reported vision loss in those over the age of 65 Activities of Daily Living needs such as housekeeping, grocery shopping, and food preparation were largely unmet [16] and Williams et al found that people with macular degeneration were more likely to need help with daily activities [17].

2.3. Impact of AMD on society

It is difficult to quantify the financial burden of AMD disease on society and there have been few studies specifically addressing this complex subject. In the UK for example, the

National Health Service (NHS) spends more than £20 billion per year on long-term, residential and home care and it can be envisaged that redirecting a fraction of this sum towards helping people maintain independence such as by the provision of inexpensive low vision aids may save billions of pounds per year [33]. Scuffham et al [34] examined the cost of injurious falls associated with visual impairment in the UK and showed that the National Health Service currently spends £1.7 billion per year treating hip fracture resulting from falls and given that older people with sight problems are more likely to fall than non-visually impaired older people this sum might be significantly reduced by attending to visual impairment. Studies have also looked at individual ocular diseases in order to quantify the cost-effectiveness of treatment verses no treatment which is an important consideration with an ever increasing financial burden of healthcare [35]. Photodynamic therapy (PDT) and the use of Anti-Vascular endothelial growth factor (VEGF) treatments have highlighted this controversy and rationing in health care has, as yet, prevented this treatment from being made available to all. Sharma et al determined the cost-effectiveness of PDT for the treatment of subfoveal choroidal neovascularisation (CNV) in patients with disciform degeneration in one eye and who's second and better-seeing eye develops visual loss secondary to predominantly classic subfoveal CNV. The authors concluded that PDT can be considered to be a treatment that is of only minimal cost-effectiveness for AMD patients who have subfoveal CNV in their second and better-seeing eyes and who have good presenting visual acuity at baseline and is a cost-ineffective treatment for AMD patients who have poor visual acuities in their affected better-seeing eyes [36]. However the same authors also examined the expected gain in quality of life-adjusted life-years (QALYs) associated with photodynamic therapy for the treatment of subfoveal CNV. Photodynamic therapy was associated with a relative increase in QALYs of 11.3% compared with placebo [36]. This example alone highlights the problems of attempting to cost quality of life.

Epidemiological data for many of the issues outlined here is often scarce and may be non-comparable between studies, however epidemiological studies remain an important tool for assessing the distribution and determinants of disease in a population and can be used to evaluate interventions.

3. Risk factors for AMD

The search for modifiable risk factors for AMD has gained impetus over the past two decades and this has largely stemmed from the development of clearer definitions of disease. The advent of appropriate grading scales [37;38], knowledge of natural history and progression and the identification of sub-types of AMD, enables comparison and corroboration of data between studies, adding weight to putative risk associations. However, some of the data can be conflicting due to the large numbers of possible risk factors assessed. Despite the limitations of these studies, there has been consensus that age, smoking and genetic make-up are risk factors for developing AMD.

3.1. Demographics

3.1.1. Age

Age is the strongest risk factor for AMD and ARM. An age of 50 yrs was taken to be the minimum criteria for the findings of drusen and other changes to be described as ARM in the International Classification System of age related maculopathy [37] and this has generally been accepted as the cut-off for defining maculopathy as being age-related. In a meta-analysis all studies found a strong association with increasing age [39]. Population studies universally show increasing prevalence with age [9;40-43]. A meta-analysis of three large population studies by Smith et al gives age-specific prevalence of sub-groups of ARM and AMD [44]. The authors reviewed the findings from the Beaver Dam, Rotterdam and Blue Mountains eye studies. All these studies used the Wisconsin grading system for ARM and AMD enabling direct comparisons between prevalence rates. The AMD lesions, namely geographic atrophy (GA) or choroidal neovascularisation (CNV) were found to have an overall prevalence of 1.63% in the populations when combined (note: the age range was from 43-99 years overall but in the analysis by Smith et al they only reviewed the data on the age range common to all three studies which was 55-86). These specific AMD lesions were not found in anyone below the age of 55 years in any of the populations. The incidence of AMD rises with age being 0.21% in those 55-64, 0.85% in those 60-74 then a dramatic rise to 4.59% in those 75-84 and 13.05% of those aged 85+ [45]. The average age at which wet AMD develops is 75 years [46]. Incidences of drusen, RPE changes, geographic atrophy, and exudative disease all increase, as exemplified by the 8- to 17-fold increased risk of developing AMD demonstrated between ages 50 and 90.

3.1.2. Gender

The evidence is conflicting for gender as a risk factor. The Beaver Dam eye study indicates both a higher incidence of early ARM in women over the age of 75(ratio 2.2:1) [2] and a higher incidence of exudative AMD in this same age group (ratio 2.6:1) [9]. This difference was not explained by selective mortality. Other studies have not been able to demonstrate this clear sex prevalence. In the Rotterdam study presence of hypo- or hyperpigmentation was higher in men but there was no difference in the sex ratio for atrophic (GA) or neovascular AMD [41]. Mitchell et al in the Blue Mountains Eye Study found consistently higher rates for AMD in women in each 10-year age-group but this difference was found not to be significant when adjusting for age in a logistic regression. They also used the same statistic on the figures from the Beaver Dam eye study using an age-adjusted relative risk of 1.27 and found the sex difference to be non-significant. Smith et al [44] found there to be no difference in the age-specific prevalence of AMD between men and women in the Beaver Dam, Rotterdam and Blue Mountains studies. Evans summarises this well and concludes that, although more studies have demonstrated a slight increased risk in women in the older age-groups, it could not be confirmed that all age-effects and health-seeking behaviours were taken into account [47]. The meta-analysis by Chakratharty et al suggests that there is no significant association between female gender and late AMD. In the case control studies included in the analysis, the overall

OR for female gender was 1.00 (95% CI 0.83 - 1.21). In the cross-sectional studies, it was 1.06 (95% CI 0.78 - 1.44) and in the prospective studies, it was 1.01 (95% CI 0.89 - 1.16) [39].

3.1.3. Ethnicity

Several studies have looked at incidence and prevalence by ethnicity and there are established differences. Comparison of the three large population studies from Holland, the US and Australia demonstrated a lower prevalence of neovascular AMD in the Dutch population [44]. All late forms of AMD appear to be more common in the White population as compared to Black and Hispanic populations [48;49]. However the highest frequency for exudative AMD appeared to be in Chinese (age- and gender-adjusted odds ratio, 4.30; 95% confidence interval, 1.30-14.27) compared with whites [50]. Choroidal melanin has been hypothesized to have a protective effect on the RPE, photoreceptors, and Bruch's membrane, perhaps through an antioxidant effect or an ability to absorb light rays that damage the posterior layers of the retina [51]. However, in most of these studies that included both whites and blacks, there were too few blacks with neovascular AMD to examine the reason for these racial differences. Although the incidence of neovascular AMD in blacks is lower, it is not negligible. Data from one recent study, the Salisbury Eye Evaluation, showed that the prevalence of choroidal neovascularization was 1.1% in blacks, compared with 1.7% in whites [52].

When examining specific features of age-related macular change, the Baltimore Eye Survey found large drusen (>125 microm), pigment abnormalities and AMD were more common among older whites compared with blacks. The prevalence of AMD was 2.1 % among whites over 70 years of age. No cases of AMD were detected among 243 black subjects in this age group [53]. In addition the spectrum of neovascular maculopathy in black Americans was found to differ from that typically seen in whites, both clinically and demographically. In a retrospective review of over 100 angiograms for AMD, CNV in blacks was more commonly juxtapapillary and more had CNV in the absence of drusen or other known predisposing conditions. Disciform-stage CNV in blacks was associated with a greater degree of pigment proliferation than that typically noted in whites. Demographically, there was a significant female predominance of CNV in blacks (87%) compared with population studies [54]. In Vancouver a total of 88 ethnic Chinese patients were identified among 10,000 angiograms. Pigment epithelial detachments were more than twice as common in the overall group of ethnic Chinese patients as in their counterparts of European ancestry (OR 2.6, 95% CI 0.7 to 10.1). The relative prevalence of the two main late AMD subtypes (GA and CNV) varies according to the population studied. In the Beaver Dam [9], Rotterdam [41] and Blue Mountains [42] eye studies the overall ratio of GA to CNV was 1:2. Whereas in the Reykjavik eye study [55] the ratio is reversed with an overall relative prevalence of GA to CNV of 4.5:1 (3: 1 in those 70+) but it was noted that a common ancestor was found in those with GA only 6 generations back compared with the norm of 12 generations in the Icelandic population. In Japan there is evidence that AMD is increasing quite dramatically which would refute the idea of a racial component to the disease and would imply that lifestyle factors may be more important. The number of exudative AMD patients in all ophthalmology departments throughout Japan was estimated to be 14,400 in 1993. This number was estimated to have almost doubled over the six year period since the initial survey in 1987 [56]. In Greenland an unusual form of AMD is described as retino-choroidal atrophy (RCA). The clinical picture of RCA is peripapillary and central retino-choroidal atrophy and sclerosis. In 1997 Ostenfeld-Akerblom et al examined 22 patients with AMD and of these 12 patients had RCA, which was the most common type of AMD in this Greenlandic investigation. All were severely visually handicapped with a visual acuity less than or equal to Snellen 6/60 [57]. Similarly, in African-Americans and Asians the pattern of disease does appear to be different with polypoidal chorio-vasculopathy (PCV) being more common [58].

3.1.4. Geography

It is difficult to separate the effects of geography from race and there is little evidence to suggest that geography per-say has an influence. However it has been shown that the prevalence in immigrants tends towards that of the native population and the assumption is that diet and lifestyle influences disease presentation [59;60].

3.1.5. Socioeconomics

It has been shown that visual impairment reflects socioeconomic status [61] and there is limited research specifically looking at the socio-demographics of people with age-related macular degeneration. However after controlling for smoking, age, sex and less vitamin supplementation Klein et al [62] found incidence of early ARM was highest in those in the service industries and blue collar workers and in those with less formal education. The association of early and late ARM with less education was also demonstrated in the AREDS study [63] and the EDCCS demonstrated an association of less education with CNV [64]. The Beijing eye study shows conflicting evidence with an early report noting early ARM was statistically associated with living in a rural region ($p<0.001$; 95% CI: 0.17 to 0.49) and lower level of education ($p = 0.01$; 95% CI: 1.07 to 1.65) [65] but a later report showing no statistical association [66]. In another Chinese study, high educational background was a protective factor for AMD (OR: 0.761, 95% CI: 0.51-0.98) [67]. However other studies have not been able to show an association [48;68-71]. The difficulty of establishing a link with socioeconomic status is that in itself it comprises many facets and confounders are thus difficult to quantify but the majority of cross-sectional studies appear to support an association with lower levels of education.

3.2. Personal characteristics

3.2.1. Hair colour / skin sun-sensitivity

Although sun-exposure might in itself be a risk for AMD, it is recognised that sun-sensitivity and sun-avoidance may be confounding factors [72]. In the case-control study by Darzins et al [73] they were able to demonstrate significantly poorer tanning ability (skin types I or II) in cases with AMD in chi-squared analysis. However, age and smoking as well as sun-exposure are all possible confounders and were not included in the analysis. Data from the Blue mountains study [72] indicated greater skin sun-sensitivity in those with AMD but also reduced skin sun-sensitivity; possibly explained by increased biological risk in those with sensitive skin but overridden by sun avoidance in those with average tanning skin and but increased sun exposure in the darker skin category. Khan et al found no association between skin sun-sensitivity and late AMD [74]. Hair colour may be associated with ocular pigmentation and has also been postulated as a possible identifiable risk factor for AMD, however no association was found in either the Blue Mountains Eye Study or the case-control study by Khan et al [72;74].

3.2.2. Iris colour

Four case-control studies have demonstrated an association between light iris colour and macular degeneration [75-78]. Three of these studies looked at cases with a broad definition of macular degeneration, which included cases of ARM as well as AMD [75-78], and all appeared to shown an association of AMD with lighter iris pigment. However, the control groups are not clearly defined in two of the studies [76;77], the studies did not always define a specific grading protocol for iris colour and did not look at potential confounding factors such as smoking and age in a logistic regression approach. Khan et al, in a study of well-defined GA and CNV with adjustment for potential confounders, showed that whilst there was a trend for lighter iris colour to be associated more frequently with geographic atrophy type AMD, this did not reach clinical significance. In a case series, Sandberg et al suggest that light iris colour may be associated with more severe neovascular AMD with more extensive retinal degeneration [79] than might occur in patients with darker irides. Holz [80] demonstrated that iris colour per-say may not be linked to ARM but that a change in iris colour with loss of stromal pigmentation may be associated with increased risk of ARM. The grouping of different phenotypes of AMD in some studies may have diluted any association of iris colour and AMD and hence it is difficult to be certain if there is any true association. Iris colour has also been explored in population studies [64] however, the numbers of late AMD may have been too small to detect any association. In the Blue Mountains eye study [72] an association was detected for blue iris colour alone when compared with all other iris colours, in both late AMD and early ARM and this was using a multiple logistic regression approach correcting for confounders of smoking, age, gender and family history of AMD. Lighter-coloured irides were associated with GA (OR, 5.0; 95% CI, 1.0, 25.3) in the Latinos Los-Angeles eye study [81]. On balance, whilst there may be a small association between lighter iris colour and AMD, the effect appears to be small and other risk factors are likely to outweigh any effect of iris pigmentation.

3.2.3. Refractive error and axial length

Several authors have demonstrated a relationship between hyperopia and AMD, more specifically CNV. Sandberg and co-workers found patients with unilateral neovascular AMD had an average spherical equivalent that was 1.0 diopter (D) more hyperopic than that of patients with the bilateral dry form. Patients with a refractive error of +0.75 D or greater were more likely to have the neovascular form compared with patients with other refractive errors [82]. A number of case-control and population cross-sectional studies also confirm an association with shorter axial length and AMD [83 63;84 85]. In the Beijing eye study, hyperopic refractive error, besides age was the single most important risk factor for ARM in adult Chinese

[65]. It is thought that hyperopia might cause secondary changes in the choroidal vasculature, predisposing them to choroidal neovascularization [86].

3.3. Genetics

The first information assessing genetic risk was demonstrated in twin and familial aggregation studies. Candidate gene studies then attempted to associate putative disease-causing polymorphisms with disease, but this relied on scarce knowledge of gene function and disease pathways. Thus initial studies examined known monogenic macular dystrophies as potential candidate genes. Non-retinal disease-causing genes then began to be explored and with the discovery of an association of APOE variants with AMD. This opened up new avenues for exploring other 'house-keeping' genes as potential candidates in AMD.

Major breakthroughs then came with family-based linkage studies of affected siblings, which identified a number of genetic loci. Thus genes known genes in these regions could be targeted and case-control association studies initially also played a role in discovering the major genetic variants for AMD. In 2010, several large-scale genome-wide association studies (GWAS) identified genes that had not been previously identified.

3.3.1. Family history and twin studies

There is strong support now for a genetic basis to AMD and ARM [87](major review). Evidence arises from a number of sources. Initially twin studies [88-92] demonstrated concordance in Monozygotic twins, greater than in dizygotic twins. Population [93-95]. There have been relatively few studies quantifying the influence of family history [75;93;94; 96-99], with estimates of the odds ratio for a positive family history conferring risk of AMD ranging from 2 to 27 [75;93;94;96;97;100].

3.3.2. Linkage studies and genome-wide association studies

Genetic linkage studies [101-103] have identified genes in large families which associate with disease. Two major disease susceptibility loci have been confirmed in a number of studies; chromosomes 1q32, which includes the gene that encodes complement factor H [CFH] and chromosome 10q26 [104;105](meta-analysis), (includes PLEKHA1, hypothetical gene LOC387715, and HTRA1). In one study genetic variation in VEGF showed evidence of linkage (HLOD = 1.32) [106] and this has been confirmed in other studies [107]. Further novel variants have been found in the TNXB-FKBPL-NOTCH4 region of chromosome 6p21 in a recent genome-wide association study and this requires further exploration.

3.3.3. Candidate gene studies

A number of autosomal genes associated with hereditary retinal dystrophies have been isolated with the majority assessed as potential candidate genes for AMD (RetNet Retinal Information Network at http://www.sph.uth.tmc.edu/retnet/). Attention has focused on those with phenotypic similarity to AMD. Stargardt disease and Best macular dystrophy commonly result in high levels of retinal pigment epithelial autofluorescence and macular atrophy.

Drusen are a prominent feature of Doyne honeycomb retinal dystrophy (autosomal dominant radial drusen; Malattia Leventinese) followed later by the development of CNV, which is also a common feature of Sorsby fundus dystrophy.

Genes associated with hereditary retinal dystrophies are not the only candidate genes for AMD. Data on environmental risk factors suggest other pathogenic processes to be explored. Positive associations have been found for proteins involved in the biological infrastructure such as the extracellular matrix [108], and the RPE [109]. Genetic polymorphisms in genes controlling angiogenesis have also been investigated [110;111]. Genes controlling lipid and cholesterol transport [112-116] have also been implicated. Apolipoprotein E (ApoE), a major lipid transporter, has two alleles of interest: ε2 and ε4. ApoE ε4 was the first gene identified that appeared to confer resistance to the disease (OR 0.43; 95% CI 0.21-0.88) [113;114]. Conversely, ApoE ε2 confers susceptibility to AMD.

The inflammation and immune response has been examined in greater detail since linkage studies revealed common variants found in complement factor H (1q) [117-119] associated with disease. CFH is a major regulator of complement cascade which is part of the innate immune system. Risk of developing AMD is associated with an allele of CFH in which a histidine residue is encoded in place of a tyrosine residue at amino acid position 402. The increased risk ranges between 2- to 4-fold for heterozygote carriers and 3- to 7-fold for homozygotes. In addition, multiple other polymorphisms, many of which are in non-coding regions of CFH or in nearby genes encoding other complement factors, demonstrate equal or stronger association with disease susceptibility than does the CFH Y402H variant [120;121 122]. No single polymorphism accounts for the entire contribution of CFH to disease susceptibility and there appears to be a number of polymorphisms, some conferring risk, others reducing risk [123;124]. At 10q26, a number of genes have been implicated. A single nucleotide polymorphism (SNP) in the promoter of the HTRA1 gene was associated with a population attributable risk of 49.3% and a 10-times greater risk of developing CNV [125]. Another susceptibility locus PLEKHA1/ LOC387715 also mapped to chromosome 10q26 [126;127]. In the study by Jakobsdottir, the association of either a single or a double copy of the high-risk allele within the PLEKHA1/LOC387715 locus accounts for an odds ratio of 5.0 (95% confidence interval 3.2-7.9) for ARM and a population attributable risk as high as 57%.

3.4. Systemic disease

Epidemiological studies have primarily investigated hypertension and hyperlipidaemia, and the clinical manifestations of CVD such as myocardial infarctions and angina [128], although some other chronic diseases have also been investigated. Although the overall number of participants in these studies is large, there may be low prevalence of end-stage cases and in the longitudinal population studies, few incident cases. Therefore the power to test for statistically significant associations is weak, unless the relative risk is very high. Failure to find associations may also be due to the insensitivity of some of the risk factor measurements or due to selective survival. Conversely, some of the relations reported may be due to chance, bias, and unadjusted confounding.

3.4.1. *Cardiovascular disease*

Risk factors for cardiovascular disease (such as age, smoking, hypertension, hypercholesterolemia, post-menopausal estrogen use, diabetes, and dietary intake of fats, alcohol and antioxidants) have been associated with AMD in some studies. This raises the possibility that the causal pathways for cardiovascular disease and AMD may share similar risk factors [129]. However, few studies have looked at cardiovascular disease as a risk factor in its own right. In one case-control study there was a statistically significant association between coronary artery disease and AMD [83], but in the prospective case-control Age-Related Eye Disease Study (AREDS) study of 776 subjects there was no increased incident AMD with mean 6.3 years follow-up with a history of angina as a measure of cardiovascular disease [130]. A large population study, the National Health and Nutrition Examination Survey (NHANES) III showed dry AMD was with myocardial infarctions in non-Hispanic white subjects [48]. Other population-based studies have not found an association [44;131-139]. A retrospective study of Medicare records investigated the relationship between AMD and myocardial infarctions, diabetes mellitus, and hypertension [140]. They used a five percent random sample of 2000 to 2003 Medicare enrolees which included 134,246 people with dry AMD and 32,788 people with wet AMD. All three diseases were associated with AMD, particularly wet AMD, and baseline AMD was significantly associated with the development of incident myocardial infarction from which they suggest the possibility of shared common antecedents between myocardial infarction and AMD.

3.4.2. *Blood pressure*

A number of population-based cross-sectional and case-control studies have found an association between systemic hypertension and AMD [63;69;83;140-143]. The relationship appears to be complex, with the association was significant only for wet AMD in two of the studies63;143 and the association became statistically non-significant when dry and wet AMD were analysed separately in another [83]. The Beaver Dam Eye Study (BDES) found that systemic hypertension was associated with incident AMD and wet AMD at 10-year follow-up [135]. There were differences noted in this study between the association of systolic and diastolic blood pressure, with systolic BP showing a positive association with both wet AMD and RPE depigmentation while diastolic BP was inversely associated with incident early ARM. An inverse relationship between systolic BP and wet AMD was reported by the Women's Health Initiative Sight Exam Ancillary Study [139]. Other case-control and population studies have not been able to detect a statistically significant relationship between AMD and hypertension which may reflect uncontrolled factors such as treatment for or duration of hypertension [44;75;130-134;136-138;144-149].

3.4.3. *Atherosclerosis*

The Atherosclerosis Risk in Communities Study (ARIC) and the Rotterdam Study have investigated relationship of atherosclerosis as a risk factor for AMD [128;133;150] using ultrasound measurements of the common carotid intima-media thickness and to assess the presence of atherosclerotic plaques. carotid artery plaque (odds ratio, 1.77; 95% confidence interval, 1.18-2.65) and focal retinal arteriolar narrowing (odds ratio, 1.79; 95% confidence interval, 1.07-2.98) were associated with retinal pigment epithelial depigmentation only in the ARIC study but no association was detected for AMD. In the Rotterdam Study atherosclerosis was noted to be associated with a 2.5 to 4.7 times increased risk of AMD [150], suggesting there may be similar pathways in the disease process or that it might directly influence pathogenesis due to altered ocular blood flow.

3.4.4. Haematological- lipids/ Inflammatory markers

Cholesterol has been found in drusen deposits [151], and dyslipidemia, being an established risk factor for atherosclerosis might also be a risk factor for AMD. Two 10-year follow-up reports of population-based cohort studies and a case-control study have found a significant association for HDL and AMD, however both protective and adverse effects have been reported. The prospective studies also found an increasing trend of elevated total/HDL cholesterol ratio with AMD, and pure geographic atrophy [135;152]. In contrast, population-based cohort studies have not demonstrated a significant association between inflammatory markers and AMD [152;153].Other biochemical risk factors for CVD that have been investigated for their association to AMD are serum lipids, fibrinogen and C-reactive protein (CRP). Fibrinogen and CRP are inflammatory biomarkers shown to predict CAD [154]. Most studies have not found any association between serum total cholesterol, HDL and LDL cholesterol, or triglyceride levels and AMD [44;48;69;132;134;141;155 156;157]. Fibrinogen was positively associated in the baseline analysis of the BMES population, however this relationship became non-significant at the 10-year follow-up [132;152]. Seddon *et al* reported that CRP was positively associated with progression of AMD in a clinic-based cohort. Similarly, cross-sectional and case-control studies have shown positive relationships [48;132;153;158]. These findings support an inflammatory aetiology for AMD pathogenesis with a minor, if at all, contribution from serum lipids.

3.4.5. Stroke

Most studies have been unable to find an association between stroke and AMD [131 132 48 44; 133;134 135;136;139]. In the ARIC study early ARM predicted incident stroke in middle-aged persons, however there were too few cases of late AMD to establish any association [159]. This finding is supported with incident early ARM predicted by stroke in the Blue mountains eye study [152]. Thus far, an association between late AMD and stroke has not been established.

3.4.6. Body mass index

There have been some positive associations noted between high BMI and early AMD. [135;139;152;160-162]. In the AREDS study, greater body mass was found to be associated with higher risk of incident GA after mean follow-up of 6.3 years [130]. Also Seddon et al specifically evaluated progression from early or intermediate AMD to advanced AMD and demonstrated an increased risk with higher BMI. [160]. However, pooled analyses of 3 large population cohort studies have found no association between BMI and AMD [44;136]. In fact, in some of these studies there has been shown an association of lean body mass with increased risk of GA

[132;135;161] this association was not found in the AREDS. It therefore appears the association is not yet universally established.

3.4.7. Diabetes

Diabetes may theoretically be a risk factor for AMD by influencing choroidal blood flow [163] and increased plasma fibrinogen which may independently be associated with AMD [132]. Associations have been made between diabetes and wet AMD in some studies [130;139;140;163]. But there is little evidence of an association with dry AMD [130, 139, 140]. Interestingly, the BMES found no association with wet AMD, but a significant relationship with dry AMD [164]. In a meta-analysis, estimates from four prospective cohort studies demonstrated the presence of diabetes to be associated with an increased risk of late AMD (RR 1.66; 95% CI 1.05 - 2.63) [147;152;165;166] and similarly meta-analysis of data from two cross-sectional studies [167] associations were non-significant (OR 1.09; 95% CI 0.61 - 1.92). One case control study [148] showed non- significant association with diabetes (OR 0.55; 95% CI 0.06 - 4.87). Certainly the evidence points to only a weak association between diabetes and AMD.

3.4.8. Other chronic diseases

Some diseases which have been postulated to have common pathogenesis with AMD include Alzheimer's disease (AD), gout and emphysema. In the Beaver Dam Eye Study, a history of emphysema at baseline was associated with the incidence of retinal pigment epithelial depigmentation (RR = 2.84; 95% CI, 1.40-5.78), increased retinal pigment (RR = 2.20; 95% CI, 1.11-4.35), and exudative macular degeneration (RR = 5.12; 95% CI, 1.63-16.06). A history of gout was associated with the incidence of pure geographic atrophy (RR = 3.48; 95% CI, 1.27-9.53) [168]. Whilst in the Rotterdam population based study, although advanced age-related maculopathy at baseline showed an increased risk of incident Alzheimer's disease (relative risk = 2.1), this risk decreased after additional adjustment for smoking and athero-sclerosis (relative risk = 1.5). In a further population study, cognitive scores were lower in those with AMD even after correcting for education although Alzheimer disease was not associated with AMD. Other investigators have looked at the relationship between the CFH Y402H polymorphism (now considered a major risk gene for AMD) and Alzheimer disease but the association in one study was null [169]. Whilst in a further study, although an increased frequency of the CFH AMD-risk polymorphism was noted in those with AD, subgroup analysis showed that the association between CFH C allele and AD was only evident for individuals carrying the APOE epsilon4 allele indicating a possible association between these genes and disease phenotypes. Conversely a Hungarian study, whilst supporting the findings of others of an association between the AMD-protective and AD-risk with APOE epsilon4, found that AMD is rare in those with AD which is logical if the ApoE is a major determinant of risk in this population.

3.5. Lifestyle

Along with identifying disease and co-morbidity as potential modifiable risk factors for AMD there has also been extensive investigation of environmental and social risk factors. Smoking is the single consistent factor identified by the majority of studies. Evaluation of dietary factors and sun-exposure has been less consistent, which may partly be due to the complexity of measuring these factors.

3.5.1. Smoking

Of the many environmental factors investigated in relation to AMD, smoking is the one most consistently found to be associated with increased risk. Several case-control and population based studies have reported odds ratios typically in the range 2–5 [44;170;171,63;64;134;144;170-174]. However this has not been completely consistent finding with a few smaller studies showing no association [69;75;83;148;175;176]. McCarty et al11 argued that total length of time of smoking was the most significant factor for development of AMD rather than pack years or current or former smoking status. However, Khan et al demonstrated that, whilst a loose definition of smoker or non-smoker did not show a statistically significant relationship with AMD, when careful calculation of pack-years of smoking was measured, this showed a strong association with both CNV and GA. Risk was also influenced by living with a smoker which highlights an important public health message in demonstrating the likely increased risk with passive smoking [177]. Stopping smoking was associated with reduced odds of AMD in this study and the risk in those who had not smoked for over 20 years was comparable to non-smokers. Studies have also shown that ceasing smoking reduces risk even in those older smokers (over age 80) [178]. In the recent Eureye study, bilateral disease was associated with increased odds of heavier smoking in the preceding 25 years [179].

Experimental evidence also supports smoking as a risk factor for AMD. The foveal region of the retina has a yellow pigmentation composed primarily of the carotenoids lutein and zeaxanthin. A variety of evidence suggests that this macular pigment protects the macula from actinic damage both passively (by screening potentially harmful short-wave light) and actively as an antioxidant (by quenching reactive oxygen species). Studies have shown that cigarette smoking depresses carotenoid concentration in the blood [180]. In a study by Hammond et al [181] macular pigment density and smoking frequency were inversely related ($r = -0.498$ $P < 0.001$) in a dose-response relationship. Smoking also has an established role in upregulating inflammatory mediators [182,183] and contains the pro-oxidant hydroquinone [184] causing further oxidative damage.

3.5.2. Sun exposure

Logically increased sun-exposure could increase the exposure of the retina to oxidative processes. In experimental studies photic injury is frequently used as a model of oxidative stress. In epidemiological studies, the measurement of sun-exposure generally relies on recall diaries so evidence from epidemiological and basic scientific investigations unfortunately gives somewhat conflicting results.

Experimental evidence to suggest sunlight as a risk factor is given by in-vitro studies. In the retina, lipofuscin is located within the pigment epithelium where it is exposed to high oxygen and visible light, a prime environment for the generation of reactive oxygen species. It has been demonstrated that retinal lipofuscin is a photo-inducible generator of reactive oxygen species and this may translate into cell damage via several mechanisms. The position of lipofuscin within the lysosome implies that irradiated lipofuscin is liable to cause oxidative damage to either the lysosomal membrane or the lysosomal enzymes. One study group found that that illumination of lipofuscin with visible light is capable of extragranular lipid peroxidation, enzyme inactivation, and protein oxidation. The authors postulate that lipofuscin may compromise retinal cell function by causing loss of lysosomal integrity and that this may be a major contributory factor to the pathology associated with retinal light damage and diseases such as age-related macular degeneration [185]. It has also been shown that lipofuscin-loaded RPE cells are considerably more sensitive to visible blue light than unloaded control cells. The loaded cells showed lysosomal membrane destabilization with ensuing leakage of lytic enzymes and eventually cell death [186]. Macular pigment, consisting of lutein and zeaxanthin, through its ability to filter light and by direct antioxidative properties, has been proposed as the most effective protective factor in the central retina ("natural sun glasses") and could be important to reduce light-induced oxidative retinal damage. The observation, that with age and especially in eyes with AMD, lower concentrations of macular pigment could be found, can be interpreted that low macular pigment concentrations may be associated with higher risk for AMD. Through dietary intake and eventually with supplementation the concentration of macular pigment can be increased, and analysis of the correlation between macular pigment and AMD may be important to characterise a possible modifiable AMD risk factor [187].

One of the first studies to examine the relationship of AMD to sun exposure was a case-controls study by Hyman et al [75] of 228 cases; no association with AMD demonstrated. A larger study of the Chesapeake Bay Waterman [176] found that even with high levels of UV-B or UV-A exposure, there was no evidence of increased risk of age-related macular degeneration [176]. However a further report from the same study calculated that compared with age-matched controls, patients with advanced age-related macular degeneration (geographic atrophy or disciform scarring) had significantly higher exposure to blue or visible light over the preceding 20 years (odds ratio, 1.36 [95% CI 1.00 to 1.85]). The data suggests that high levels of exposure to blue or visible light may cause ocular damage, especially later in life, and may be related to the development of age-related macular degeneration [188]. Cross-sectional data from the BDES also suggests that the amount of leisure time spent outdoors in summer was significantly associated with exudative macular degeneration (OR, 2.26; 95% CI, 1.06 to 4.81) and late maculopathy (OR, 2.19; 95% CI, 1.12 to 4.25). Whereas, wearing eyeglasses was inversely associated with increased retinal pigment and the use of hats and sunglasses was inversely associated with soft indistinct drusen [189]. Data from the Blue Mountains Eye Study [72] indicated increased risk of late AMD associated with both high (OR, 2.54) and low (OR, 2.18) skin sun sensitivity; possibly explained by increased biological risk in those with sensitive skin but increased sun-exposure in the darker skin category. It was postulated that there may be significant confounding by skin sensitivity and sun avoidance.

No support was found for sunlight exposure as a risk factor for AMD in several other case-control studies [64;73;74;144;167]. Subjects In the POLA Study who had used sunglasses regularly had a decreased risk of soft drusen (OR = 0.81; 95% CI, 0.66-1.00) but the study did not support a deleterious effect of sunlight exposure in ARMD [167]. In a study of 3271 people in 9 randomly selected urban clusters and 4 randomly selected rural clusters in Victoria, Australia, lifetime sunlight exposure and UV-B exposure was not associated with AMD [144]. In the Newcastle (Australia) study, after stratifying by tanning ability, the median annual sun exposure of control subjects exceeded that of cases and after adjusting for age and sun-sensitivity sun-exposure was negatively associated with AMD. The authors concluded that sun-sensitivity confounds study of the postulated AMD-sunlight link [73]. The evidence is thus still lacking to support a definite link between AMD and sun-exposure.

3.5.3. Micronutrients

A significant role for vitamin C in the retina has been indicated by laboratory experiments in animals. Tso et al showed that under conditions of continuous light exposure, the levels of ascorbic acid in the retina fell [190]. The same group also demonstrated that ascorbic acid may protect the retina from light damage [191]. Retinal degeneration can be induced specifically by anti-oxidant (E and A) vitamin deficiency in monkeys [192]. Zinc is found in high concentrations in the RPE and pathological lesions have been observed in animals deprived of zinc [193]. Vitamin E and selenium play key roles in preventing in vitro lipid peroxidation and free radical damage to retinal tissues. Rats fed on diets deficient in vitamin E and/or selenium and subsequently exposed to hyperbaric oxygen show diminished ERG amplitudes and evidence of photoreceptor cell necrosis [194]. Carotenoids are vegetable products which are essential to the health of the eye and are concentrated at the macula- in particular zeaxanthin (found mainly in maize) and lutein (found mainly in spinach); they may also act as anti-oxidants to scavenge free radicals.

In light of these experimental findings the EDCCS examined the relationship of micronutrients to neovascular age-related macular degeneration [64;195]. Serum levels of carotenoids (Lutein/ Zeaxanthin, beta-carotene, alpha-carotene, cryptoxanthin, lycopene), vitamins C and E, selenium (glutathione peroxidase is selenium dependent and theoretically may reduce the amount of macular damage from oxidative insult) and zinc in 421 patients with neovascular age-related macular degeneration and 615 controls were compared. Although no statistically significant protective effect was found for vitamin C or E or selenium individually, an antioxidant index that combined all four micronutrient measurements showed statistically significant reductions of risk with increasing levels of the index. No support was found for serum zinc levels as a risk factor for neovascular AMD. In a further report dietary intake was examined in this same study group using food frequency questionnaires. A higher dietary intake of carotenoids was associated with a 43% lower risk for AMD. Lutein and zeaxanthin were most strongly associated [196].

Other population studies have not been able to demonstrate a protective effect of the antioxidant micronutrients. In the Beaver Dam Eye Study a protective effect of higher zinc intake in early but not late ARM was demonstrated but there was no association with intake of other antioxidant micronutrients [197]. The study's main failing may have been with the use of diet recall from 10 years prior; hence recall bias is likely to be a major factor limiting the ability to detect an association. Similarly the third national health and nutrition examination survey study did not find a link with serum levels of lutein/ zeaxanthin or dietary intake and AMD in the sample as a whole but only in those with young onset AMD [198]. Again recall bias is likely to be a major factor influencing the likelihood of detecting an association.

Results from a large clinical trial have indicated that high-dose vitamin supplementation may reduce vision loss from AMD [199]. The Age-related Eye Disease Study Research Group developed a double-masked clinical trial in patients with AMD. Treatment with zinc with or without antioxidant vitamins reduced the risk of progression to advanced AMD in the groups with more severe AMD at the outset (more specifically these groups were those with extensive intermediate-sized drusen, large drusen or non-central GA in one or both eyes, or advanced AMD in one eye). Relative risk estimates suggest a reduced risk of 21% if zinc is taken alone and 17% for antioxidants the reduced risk if both are taken is 25%. In the less severe AMD groups at outset the incidence of progression to advanced AMD at 5 years was too low to establish any effect of supplementation and there was no effect of supplementation on delaying progression from the less severe groups to more severe groups during the study.

At the time of writing, a multi-center, randomized trial of supplementation with Lutein, Zeaxanthin, and Omega-3 Long-Chain Polyunsaturated Fatty Acids (the AREDS 2 study) is underway, with results expected in 2013 [200].

3.5.4. Dietary fat

The major drusen component is neutral lipid and this is also deposited in Bruch's membrane. Theories therefore propose AMD as having a similar pathway to atherosclerosis. However, since the lipid is esterified, it implies the fat arises secondary to being transported out of RPE cells and does not arise from plasma cholesterol. By contrast, the lipoprotein constituent of drusen is plasma derived. There are epidemiological studies to support this theory. In one study dietary linoleic acid (the major fatty-acid component of drusen [151]) was associated with increased risk of AMD [201]. Generally the epidemiological studies show conflicting results for dietary fat which may be in part due to the difficulty inherent in food-frequency questionnaires and associated recall bias or may be further evidence that there is no association as might be expected from the underlying biology. There appears to be limited evidence for an association between saturated fatty acid intake and AMD [202]. Seddon *et al* suggest an increased risk of AMD prevalence and progression with higher vegetable fat intake [203;204], and it is hypothesised that this may be due to high levels of trans-fatty acids in some margarines. Whilst in the BMES there was a reduction of incident AMD with increasing intake of polyunsaturated fats after 5 years follow-up [205]. Omega-3 fatty acids may protect against AMD [206;207] and the AREDS2 study is currently underway to further investigate this [200].

3.5.5. Alcohol

There is experimental evidence to suggest alcohol may increase the risk of AMD. A study of alcohol-fed rats showed that heavy alcohol intake was associated with both an increased accumulation of ethyl esters in the choroid and an exacerbation of the CNV induced by laser treatment [208]. A number of clinical studies have investigated the role of alcohol consumption and risk of AMD and among these there are studies demonstrating no association [209-211], weak positive associations for some forms of ARM/ AMD [212-217], or even an inverse association [146;218]. In a recent systematic review of the literature pooled results showed that heavy alcohol consumption was associated with an increased risk of early AMD (pooled odds ratio, 1.47; 95% confidence interval, 1.10 to 1.95), whereas the association between heavy alcohol consumption and risk of late AMD was inconclusive. There were insufficient data to evaluate a dose-response association between alcohol consumption and AMD or the association between moderate alcohol consumption and AMD. The authors conclude that although this association seems to be independent of smoking, residual confounding effects from smoking cannot be excluded completely [219].

4. Summary

AMD creates a huge burden on society, being the third largest cause of blindness world-wide. The impact is far reaching in terms of quality of life to the individual as well as financial and social burdens on society as a whole. AMD appears to have greater representation in white, Caucasian populations but it is becoming apparent that the prevalence in other ethnic populations is substantial. There are differences in the sub-type presentation of disease in different populations.

It appears that AMD is caused by environmental factors triggering disease in genetically susceptible individuals. Identifying modifiable risk factors is a vital part of defining the pathogenesis of AMD and enabling appropriate targeting of treatment strategies. Whilst age is the strongest risk factor for AMD, a number of environmental risk factors have been proposed and the adverse effect of smoking is well-established.

The data demonstrate a clear association between the risk of AMD and pack-years of cigarette smoking with odds ratios in some studies demonstrating a dose-related effect. Both types of AMD show a similar relationship in most studies. Stopping smoking is associated with reduced odds of AMD. This provides strong support for a causal relationship between smoking and age-related macular degeneration. Axial length and refractive error also appear to play a role with most studies indicating increased prevalence associated with hyperopia. Other possible risk factors include blue iris colour, poor skin tanning or abnormal skin sensitivity to sunlight but generally the studies show null or only weak association. Hypertension and other cardiovascular risk factors do seem to play a role but the associations appear weaker than for smoking and genetic factors. Dietary factors associations are notoriously difficult to establish but in general there appears to be reduced risk in those with diets higher in antioxidants and fish but there is only weak evidence for an association with increased dietary fat intake. Dietary antioxidant supplements such as carotenoids and zinc may be protective for progression in the later stages of AMD and other dietary supplements are currently being investigated.

Genes associated with hereditary retinal dystrophies have been isolated but few appear to show association with AMD. However, non-retina specific genes appear to be significantly associated with risk, in particular those involved in complement activation, extracellular matrix composition, angiogenesis and lipid transport which provides vital evidence for developing targeted therapy.

Author details

Jane Khan[1,2,3,4]

1 Centre for Ophthalmology and Visual Science, University of Western Australia, Australia

2 Royal Perth Hospital, Western Australia, Australia

3 Department of Medical Technology and Physics, Sir Charles Gairdner Hospital, Perth, Western Australia, Australia

4 Western Eye, Perth, Western Australia, Australia

References

[1] Mitchell, P, Wang, J. J, Foran, S, & Smith, W. Five-year incidence of age-related maculopathy lesions: the Blue Mountains Eye Study. *Ophthalmology* (2002). , 109, 1092-7.

[2] Klein, R, Klein, B. E, Jensen, S. C, & Meuer, S. M. The five-year incidence and progression of age-related maculopathy: the Beaver Dam Eye Study. *Ophthalmology* (1997). , 104, 7-21.

[3] Van Leeuwen, R, Klaver, C. C, Vingerling, J. R, Hofman, A, & De Jong, P. T. The risk and natural course of age-related maculopathy: follow-up at 6 1/2 years in the Rotterdam study. *Arch.Ophthalmol.* (2003). , 121, 519-26.

[4] Bressler, N. M, Munoz, B, Maguire, M. G, Vitale, S. E, Schein, O. D, Taylor, H. R, et al. Five-year incidence and disappearance of drusen and retinal pigment epithelial abnormalities. Waterman study. *Arch.Ophthalmol.* (1995). , 113, 301-8.

[5] Five-year follow-up of fellow eyes of patients with age-related macular degeneration and unilateral extrafoveal choroidal neovascularizationMacular Photocoagulation Study Group. *Arch Ophthalmol* (1993). , 111, 1189-99.

[6] Gregor, Z, Bird, A. C, & Chisholm, I. H. Senile disciform macular degeneration in the second eye. *Br.J.Ophthalmol.* (1977). , 61, 141-7.

[7] Bruce I MAWEBlind and partially sighted adults in Britain: the RNIB survey. *London HSMO* (1991).

[8] Evans, J. R. Causes of blindness and partial sight in England and Wales *Studies on medical and population subjects* (1995). , 1990-1991.

[9] Klein, R, Klein, B. E, & Linton, K. L. Prevalence of age-related maculopathy. The Beaver Dam Eye Study. *Ophthalmology* (1992). , 99, 933-43.

[10] Bressler, N. M, & Bressler, S. B. Preventative ophthalmology. Age-related macular degeneration. *Ophthalmology* (1995). , 102, 1206-11.

[11] Evans, J, & Wormald, R. Is the incidence of registrable age-related macular degeneration increasing? *Br.J.Ophthalmol.* (1996). , 80, 9-14.

[12] Lee, H. K, & Scudds, R. J. Comparison of balance in older people with and without visual impairment. *Age Ageing* (2003). , 32, 643-9.

[13] Mccarty, C. A, Nanjan, M. B, & Taylor, H. R. Vision impairment predicts 5 year mortality. *Br.J Ophthalmol* (2001). , 85, 322-6.

[14] Thompson, J. R, Gibson, J. M, & Jagger, C. The association between visual impairment and mortality in elderly people. *Age Ageing* (1989). , 18, 83-8.

[15] Borger, P. H, Van Leeuwen, R, Hulsman, C. A, Wolfs, R. C, Van Der Kuip, D. A, Hofman, A, et al. Is there a direct association between age-related eye diseases and mortality? The Rotterdam Study. *Ophthalmology* (2003). , 110, 1292-6.

[16] Branch, L. G, Horowitz, A, & Carr, C. The implications for everyday life of incident self-reported visual decline among people over age 65 living in the community. *Gerontologist* (1989). , 29, 359-65.

[17] Williams, R. A, Brody, B. L, Thomas, R. G, Kaplan, R. M, & Brown, S. I. The psychosocial impact of macular degeneration. *Arch.Ophthalmol.* (1998). , 116, 514-20.

[18] Mitchell, J, Bradley, P, Anderson, S. J, Ffytche, T, & Bradley, C. Perceived quality of health care in macular disease: a survey of members of the Macular Disease Society. *Br.J Ophthalmol* (2002). , 86, 777-81.

[19] Mitchell, J, & Bradley, C. Psychometric evaluation of the 12-item Well-being Questionnaire for use with people with macular disease. *Qual.Life Res.* (2001). , 10, 465-73.

[20] Lee, P. P, Spritzer, K, & Hays, R. D. The impact of blurred vision on functioning and well-being. *Ophthalmology* (1997). , 104, 390-6.

[21] Carabellese, C, Appollonio, I, Rozzini, R, Bianchetti, A, Frisoni, G. B, Frattola, L, et al. Sensory impairment and quality of life in a community elderly population. *J.Am.Geriatr.Soc.* (1993). , 41, 401-7.

[22] Frost, N. A, Sparrow, J. M, Durant, J. S, Donovan, J. L, Peters, T. J, & Brookes, S. T. Development of a questionnaire for measurement of vision-related quality of life. *Ophthalmic Epidemiol.* (1998). , 5, 185-210.

[23] Frost, A, Eachus, J, Sparrow, J, Peters, T. J, Hopper, C, Davey-smith, G, et al. Vision-related quality of life impairment in an elderly UK population: associations with age, sex, social class and material deprivation. *Eye* (2001). , 15, 739-44.

[24] Prudham, D, & Evans, J. G. Factors associated with falls in the elderly: a community study. *Age Ageing* (1981). , 10, 141-6.

[25] Tinetti, M. E, Speechley, M, & Ginter, S. F. Risk factors for falls among elderly persons living in the community. *N.Engl.J.Med.* (1988). , 319, 1701-7.

[26] Lord, S. R, Clark, R. D, & Webster, I. W. Visual acuity and contrast sensitivity in relation to falls in an elderly population. *Age Ageing* (1991). , 20, 175-81.

[27] Lord, S. R, Sambrook, P. N, Gilbert, C, Kelly, P. J, Nguyen, T, Webster, I. W, et al. Postural stability, falls and fractures in the elderly: results from the Dubbo Osteoporosis Epidemiology Study. *Med.J.Aust.* (1994). , 160, 684-91.

[28] Tobis, J. S, Reinsch, S, Swanson, J. M, Byrd, M, & Scharf, T. Visual perception dominance of fallers among community-dwelling older adults. *J.Am.Geriatr.Soc.* (1985). , 33, 330-3.

[29] Cummings, S. R, Nevitt, M. C, Browner, W. S, Stone, K, Fox, K. M, Ensrud, K. E, et al. Risk factors for hip fracture in white women. Study of Osteoporotic Fractures Research Group. *N.Engl.J.Med.* (1995). , 332, 767-73.

[30] Ivers, R. Q, Cumming, R. G, & Mitchell, P. Visual impairment and risk of falls and fracture. *Inj.Prev.* (2002).

[31] Campbell, M. K, Bush, T. L, & Hale, W. E. Medical conditions associated with driving cessation in community-dwelling, ambulatory elders. *J.Gerontol.* (1993). SS234., 230.

[32] Owsley, C. Vision and driving in the elderly. *Optom.Vis.Sci.* (1994). , 71, 727-35.

[33] Philp, I. Developing a National Service Framework for older people. *J Epidemiol Community Health* (2002). , 56, 841-2.

[34] Scuffham, P, Chaplin, S, & Legood, R. Incidence and costs of unintentional falls in older people in the United Kingdom. *J Epidemiol Community Health* (2003). , 57, 740-4.

[35] Brown, G. C, Brown, M. M, Sharma, S, Busbee, B, & Landy, J. A cost-utility analysis of interventions for severe proliferative vitreoretinopathy. *Am J Ophthalmol* (2002). , 133, 365-72.

[36] Sharma, S, Brown, G. C, Brown, M. M, Hollands, H, & Shah, G. K. The cost-effectiveness of photodynamic therapy for fellow eyes with subfoveal choroidal neovasculari-

zation secondary to age-related macular degeneration. *Ophthalmology* (2001). , 108, 2051-9.

[37] Bird, A. C, Bressler, N. M, Bressler, S. B, Chisholm, I. H, Coscas, G, Davis, M. D, et al. An international classification and grading system for age-related maculopathy and age-related macular degeneration. The International ARM Epidemiological Study Group. *Surv.Ophthalmol.* (1995). , 39, 367-74.

[38] Klein, R, Davis, M. D, Magli, Y. L, Segal, P, Klein, B. E, & Hubbard, L. The Wisconsin age-related maculopathy grading system. *Ophthalmology* (1991). , 98, 1128-34.

[39] Chakravarthy, U, Wong, T. Y, Fletcher, A, Piault, E, Evans, C, Zlateva, G, et al. Clinical risk factors for age-related macular degeneration: a systematic review and meta-analysis. *BMC.Ophthalmol.* (2010).

[40] Kini, M. M, Leibowitz, H. M, Colton, T, Nickerson, R. J, Ganley, J, & Dawber, T. R. Prevalence of senile cataract, diabetic retinopathy, senile macular degeneration, and open-angle glaucoma in the Framingham eye study. *Am.J.Ophthalmol.* (1978). , 85, 28-34.

[41] Vingerling, J. R, Dielemans, I, Hofman, A, Grobbee, D. E, Hijmering, M, Kramer, C. F, et al. The prevalence of age-related maculopathy in the Rotterdam Study. *Ophthalmology* (1995). , 102, 205-10.

[42] Mitchell, P, Smith, W, Attebo, K, & Wang, J. J. Prevalence of age-related maculopathy in Australia. The Blue Mountains Eye Study. *Ophthalmology* (1995). , 102, 1450-60.

[43] Vannewkirk, M. R, Nanjan, M. B, Wang, J. J, Mitchell, P, Taylor, H. R, & Mccarty, C. A. The prevalence of age-related maculopathy: the visual impairment project. *Ophthalmology* (2000). , 107, 1593-600.

[44] Smith, W, Assink, J, Klein, R, Mitchell, P, Klaver, C. C, Klein, B. E, et al. Risk factors for age-related macular degeneration: Pooled findings from three continents. *Ophthalmology* (2001). , 108, 697-704.

[45] Van Leeuwen, R, Klaver, C. C, Vingerling, J. R, Hofman, A, & De Jong, P. T. Epidemiology of age-related maculopathy: a review. *Eur.J Epidemiol* (2003). , 18, 845-54.

[46] Pauleikhoff, D. neovascular age-related macular degeneration: Natural History and Treatment Outcomes. *Retina* (2005). , 25, 1065-84.

[47] Evans, J. R. Risk factors for age-related macular degeneration. *Prog.Retin.Eye Res.* (2001). , 20, 227-53.

[48] Klein, R, Klein, B. E, Jensen, S. C, Mares-perlman, J. A, Cruickshanks, K. J, & Palta, M. Age-related maculopathy in a multiracial United States population: the National Health and Nutrition Examination Survey III. *Ophthalmology* (1999). , 106, 1056-65.

[49] Cruickshanks, K. J, Hamman, R. F, Klein, R, Nondahl, D. M, & Shetterly, S. M. The prevalence of age-related maculopathy by geographic region and ethnicity. The Col-

orado-Wisconsin Study of Age-Related Maculopathy. *Arch.Ophthalmol.* (1997). , 115, 242-50.

[50] Klein, R, Klein, B. E, Knudtson, M. D, Wong, T. Y, Cotch, M. F, Liu, K, et al. Prevalence of age-related macular degeneration in 4 racial/ethnic groups in the multi-ethnic study of atherosclerosis. *Ophthalmology* (2006). , 113, 373-80.

[51] Hageman, G. S, & Luthert, P. J. Victor Chong NH, Johnson LV, Anderson DH, Mullins RF. An integrated hypothesis that considers drusen as biomarkers of immune-mediated processes at the RPE-Bruch's membrane interface in aging and age-related macular degeneration. *Prog.Retin.Eye Res.* (2001). , 20, 705-32.

[52] Chang, M. A, Bressler, S. B, Munoz, B, & West, S. K. Racial differences and other risk factors for incidence and progression of age-related macular degeneration: Salisbury Eye Evaluation (SEE) Project. *Invest Ophthalmol.Vis.Sci.* (2008). , 49, 2395-402.

[53] Friedman, D. S, Katz, J, Bressler, N. M, Rahmani, B, & Tielsch, J. M. Racial differences in the prevalence of age-related macular degeneration: the Baltimore Eye Survey. *Ophthalmology* (1999). , 106, 1049-55.

[54] Capone, A. Jr., Wallace RT, Meredith TA. Symptomatic choroidal neovascularization in blacks. *Arch.Ophthalmol* (1994). , 112, 1091-7.

[55] Jonasson, F, Arnarsson, A, Sasaki, H, Peto, T, Sasaki, K, & Bird, A. C. The prevalence of age-related maculopathy in iceland: Reykjavik eye study. *Arch Ophthalmol* (2003). , 121, 379-85.

[56] Tamakoshi, A, Yuzawa, M, Matsui, M, Uyama, M, Fujiwara, N. K, & Ohno, Y. Smoking and neovascular form of age related macular degeneration in late middle aged males: findings from a case-control study in Japan. Research Committee on Chorioretinal Degenerations. *Br.J.Ophthalmol.* (1997). , 81, 901-4.

[57] Ostenfeld-akerblom, A. Age-related macular degeneration in Inuit. *Acta Ophthalmol.Scand.* (1999). , 77, 76-8.

[58] Ciardella, A. P, Donsoff, I. M, Huang, S. J, Costa, D. L, & Yannuzzi, L. A. Polypoidal choroidal vasculopathy. *Surv.Ophthalmol.* (2004). , 49, 25-37.

[59] TabaOguido APMPrevalence of age-relatd macular degeneration in Japanese immigrants living in Londrina (PR)- Brazil. *Arq Bras.Oftalmol.* (2008). , 71, 375-80.

[60] Pagliarini, S, Moramarco, A, Wormald, R. P, Piguet, B, Carresi, C, Balacco-gabrieli, C, et al. Age-related macular disease in rural southern Italy. *Arch.Ophthalmol.* (1997). , 115, 616-22.

[61] Tielsch, J. M, Sommer, A, Katz, J, Quigley, H, & Ezrine, S. Socioeconomic status and visual impairment among urban Americans. Baltimore Eye Survey Research Group. *Arch.Ophthalmol.* (1991). , 109, 637-41.

[62] Klein, R, Klein, B. E, Jensen, S. C, & Moss, S. E. The relation of socioeconomic factors to the incidence of early age-related maculopathy: the Beaver Dam eye study. *Am J Ophthalmol* (2001)., 132, 128-31.

[63] Risk factors associated with age-related macular degenerationA case-control study in the age-related eye disease study: age-related eye disease study report Age-Related Eye Disease Study Research Group. *Ophthalmology* (2000)., 107(3), 2224-32.

[64] Risk factors for neovascular age-related macular degenerationThe Eye Disease Case-Control Study Group. *Arch Ophthalmol* (1992)., 110, 1701-8.

[65] Xu, L, Li, Y, Zheng, Y, & Jonas, J. B. Associated factors for age related maculopathy in the adult population in China: the Beijing eye study. *Br.J.Ophthalmol.* (2006)., 90, 1087-90.

[66] Xu, L, Wang, Y. X, & Jonas, J. B. Level of education associated with ophthalmic diseases. The Beijing Eye Study. *Graefes Arch.Clin.Exp.Ophthalmol.* (2010)., 248, 49-57.

[67] Jia, L, Shen, X, Fan, R, Sun, Y, Pan, X, Yanh, H, et al. Risk factors for age-related macular degeneration in elderly Chinese population in Shenyang of China. *Biomed.Environ.Sci.* (2011)., 24, 506-11.

[68] Klein, R, Klein, B. E, Jensen, S. C, Moss, S. E, & Cruickshanks, K. J. The relation of socioeconomic factors to age-related cataract, maculopathy, and impaired vision. The Beaver Dam Eye Study. *Ophthalmology* (1994)., 101, 1969-79.

[69] Kahn, H. A, Leibowitz, H. M, Ganley, J. P, Kini, M. M, Colton, T, Nickerson, R. S, et al. The Framingham Eye Study. I. Outline and major prevalence findings. *Am.J.Epidemiol.* (1977)., 106, 17-32.

[70] Deangelis, M. M, Lane, A. M, Shah, C. P, Ott, J, Dryja, T. P, & Miller, J. W. Extremely discordant sib-pair study design to determine risk factors for neovascular age-related macular degeneration. *Arch.Ophthalmol.* (2004)., 122, 575-80.

[71] Attebo, K, Mitchell, P, & Smith, W. Visual acuity and the causes of visual loss in Australia. The Blue Mountains Eye Study. *Ophthalmology* (1996)., 103, 357-64.

[72] Mitchell, P, Smith, W, & Wang, J. J. Iris color, skin sun sensitivity, and age-related maculopathy. The Blue Mountains Eye Study. *Ophthalmology* (1998)., 105, 1359-63.

[73] Darzins, P, Mitchell, P, & Heller, R. F. Sun exposure and age-related macular degeneration. An Australian case-control study. *Ophthalmology* (1997)., 104, 770-6.

[74] Khan, J. C, Shahid, H, Thurlby, D. A, Bradley, M, Clayton, D. G, Moore, A. T, et al. Age related macular degeneration and sun exposure, iris colour, and skin sensitivity to sunlight. *Br.J.Ophthalmol.* (2006)., 90, 29-32.

[75] Hyman, L. G, Lilienfeld, A. M, & Ferris, F. L. III, Fine SL. Senile macular degeneration: a case-control study. *Am.J.Epidemiol.* (1983)., 118, 213-27.

[76] Weiter, J. J, Delori, F. C, Wing, G. L, & Fitch, K. A. Relationship of senile macular degeneration to ocular pigmentation. *Am J Ophthalmol* (1985)., 99, 185-7.

[77] Frank, R. N, Puklin, J. E, Stock, C, & Canter, L. A. Race, iris color, and age-related macular degeneration. *Trans.Am.Ophthalmol Soc.* (2000)., 98, 109-15.

[78] Khan, J. C, Shahid, H, Thurlby, D. A, Bradley, M, Clayton, D. G, Moore, A. T, et al. Age related macular degeneration and sun exposure, iris colour, and skin sensitivity to sunlight. *Br.J.Ophthalmol.* (2006)., 90, 29-32.

[79] Sandberg, M. A, Gaudio, A. R, Miller, S, & Weiner, A. Iris pigmentation and extent of disease in patients with neovascular age-related macular degeneration. *Invest Ophthalmol.Vis.Sci.* (1994)., 35, 2734-40.

[80] Holz, F. G, Piguet, B, Minassian, D. C, Bird, A. C, & Weale, R. A. Decreasing stromal iris pigmentation as a risk factor for age-related macular degeneration. *Am J Ophthalmol* (1994)., 117, 19-23.

[81] Fraser-bell, S, Choudhury, F, Klein, R, Azen, S, & Varma, R. Ocular risk factors for age-related macular degeneration: the Los Angeles Latino Eye Study. *Am.J.Ophthalmol.* (2010)., 149, 735-40.

[82] Sandberg, M. A, Tolentino, M. J, Miller, S, Berson, E. L, & Gaudio, A. R. Hyperopia and neovascularization in age-related macular degeneration. *Ophthalmology* (1993)., 100, 1009-13.

[83] Chaine, G, Hullo, A, Sahel, J, Soubrane, G, Espinasse-berrod, M. A, Schutz, D, et al. Case-control study of the risk factors for age related macular degeneration. France-DMLA Study Group. *Br.J Ophthalmol* (1998)., 82, 996-1002.

[84] Ikram, M. K, Van Leeuwen, R, Vingerling, J. R, Hofman, A, & De Jong, P. T. Relationship between refraction and prevalent as well as incident age-related maculopathy: the Rotterdam Study. *Invest Ophthalmol Vis.Sci.* (2003)., 44, 3778-82.

[85] Fraser-bell, S, Choudhury, F, Klein, R, Azen, S, & Varma, R. Ocular risk factors for age-related macular degeneration: the Los Angeles Latino Eye Study. *Am.J.Ophthalmol.* (2010)., 149, 735-40.

[86] Boker, T, Fang, T, & Steinmetz, R. Refractive error and choroidal perfusion characteristics in patients with choroidal neovascularization and age-related macular degeneration. *Ger J.Ophthalmol.* (1993)., 2, 10-3.

[87] Haddad, S, Chen, C. A, Santangelo, S. L, & Seddon, J. M. The genetics of age-related macular degeneration: a review of progress to date. *Surv.Ophthalmol.* (2006)., 51, 316-63.

[88] Klein, M. L, Mauldin, W. M, & Stoumbos, V. D. Heredity and age-related macular degeneration. Observations in monozygotic twins. *Arch.Ophthalmol.* (1994)., 112, 932-7.

[89] Hammond, B. R. Jr., Fuld K, Curran-Celentano J. Macular pigment density in monozygotic twins. *Invest Ophthalmol.Vis.Sci.* (1995)., 36, 2531-41.

[90] Gottfredsdottir, M. S, Sverrisson, T, Musch, D. C, & Stefansson, E. Age related macular degeneration in monozygotic twins and their spouses in Iceland. *Acta Ophthalmol Scand.* (1999)., 77, 422-5.

[91] Meyers, S. M, Greene, T, & Gutman, F. A. A twin study of age-related macular degeneration. *Am.J.Ophthalmol.* (1995)., 120, 757-66.

[92] Hammond, C. J, Webster, A. R, Snieder, H, Bird, A. C, Gilbert, C. E, & Spector, T. D. Genetic influence on early age-related maculopathy: a twin study. *Ophthalmology* (2002)., 109, 730-6.

[93] Smith, W, & Mitchell, P. Family history and age-related maculopathy: the Blue Mountains Eye Study. *Aust.N.Z.J Ophthalmol* (1998)., 26, 203-6.

[94] Klaver, C. C, Wolfs, R. C, Assink, J. J, Van Duijn, C. M, Hofman, A, & De Jong, P. T. Genetic risk of age-related maculopathy. Population-based familial aggregation study. *Arch Ophthalmol* (1998)., 116, 1646-51.

[95] Heiba, I. M, Elston, R. C, Klein, B. E, & Klein, R. Sibling correlations and segregation analysis of age-related maculopathy: the Beaver Dam Eye Study. *Genet.Epidemiol.* (1994)., 11, 51-67.

[96] Silvestri, G, Johnston, P. B, & Hughes, A. E. Is genetic predisposition an important risk factor in age-related macular degeneration? *Eye* (1994). Pt 5):564-8.

[97] Seddon, J. M, Ajani, U. A, & Mitchell, B. D. Familial aggregation of age-related maculopathy. *Am.J.Ophthalmol.* (1997)., 123, 199-206.

[98] Klein, B. E, Klein, R, Lee, K. E, Moore, E. L, & Danforth, L. Risk of incident age-related eye diseases in people with an affected sibling : The Beaver Dam Eye Study. *Am J Epidemiol.* (2001)., 154, 207-11.

[99] Piguet, B, Wells, J. A, Palmvang, I. B, Wormald, R, Chisholm, I. H, & Bird, A. C. Age-related Bruch's membrane change: a clinical study of the relative role of heredity and environment. *Br.J.Ophthalmol.* (1993)., 77, 400-3.

[100] Shahid, H, Khan, J. C, Cipriani, V, Sepp, T, Matharu, B. K, Bunce, C, et al. Age-related macular degeneration: the importance of family history as a risk factor. *Br.J.Ophthalmol.* (2012)., 96, 427-31.

[101] Klein, M. L, Schultz, D. W, Edwards, A, Matise, T. C, Rust, K, Berselli, C. B, et al. Age-related macular degeneration. Clinical features in a large family and linkage to chromosome 1q. *Arch.Ophthalmol.* (1998)., 116, 1082-8.

[102] Weeks, D. E, Conley, Y. P, Tsai, H. J, Mah, T. S, Rosenfeld, P. J, Paul, T. O, et al. Age-related maculopathy: an expanded genome-wide scan with evidence of susceptibility loci within the 1q31 and 17q25 regions. *Am J Ophthalmol* (2001)., 132, 682-92.

[103] Schultz, D. W, Klein, M. L, Humpert, A. J, Luzier, C. W, Persun, V, Schain, M, et al. Analysis of the ARMD1 locus: evidence that a mutation in HEMICENTIN-1 is associated with age-related macular degeneration in a large family. *Hum.Mol.Genet.* (2003). , 12, 3315-23.

[104] Majewski, J, Schultz, D. W, Weleber, R. G, Schain, M. B, Edwards, A. O, Matise, T. C, et al. Age-related macular degeneration--a genome scan in extended families. *Am.J Hum.Genet.* (2003). , 73, 540-50.

[105] Fisher, S. A, Abecasis, G. R, Yashar, B. M, Zareparsi, S, Swaroop, A, Iyengar, S. K, et al. Meta-analysis of genome scans of age-related macular degeneration. *Hum.Mol.Genet.* (2005). , 14, 2257-64.

[106] Haines, J. L, Schnetz-boutaud, N, Schmidt, S, Scott, W. K, Agarwal, A, Postel, E. A, et al. Functional candidate genes in age-related macular degeneration: significant association with VEGF, VLDLR, and LRP6. *Invest Ophthalmol.Vis.Sci.* (2006). , 47, 329-35.

[107] Churchill, A. J, Carter, J. G, Lovell, H. C, Ramsden, C, Turner, S. J, Yeung, A, et al. VEGF polymorphisms are associated with neovascular age-related macular degeneration. *Hum.Mol.Genet.* (2006). , 15, 2955-61.

[108] Johnson, L. V, & Anderson, D. H. Age-related macular degeneration and the extracellular matrix. *N.Engl.J Med.* (2004). , 351, 320-2.

[109] Zurdel, J, Finckh, U, Menzer, G, Nitsch, R. M, & Richard, G. CST3 genotype associated with exudative age related macular degeneration. *Br.J Ophthalmol* (2002). , 86, 214-9.

[110] Fiotti, N, Pedio, M, Battaglia, P. M, Altamura, N, Uxa, L, Guarnieri, G, et al. MMP-9 microsatellite polymorphism and susceptibility to exudative form of age-related macular degeneration. *Genet.Med.* (2005). , 7, 272-7.

[111] Haines, J. L, Schnetz-boutaud, N, Schmidt, S, Scott, W. K, Agarwal, A, Postel, E. A, et al. Functional candidate genes in age-related macular degeneration: significant association with VEGF, VLDLR, and LRP6. *Invest Ophthalmol.Vis.Sci.* (2006). , 47, 329-35.

[112] Conley, Y. P, Thalamuthu, A, Jakobsdottir, J, Weeks, D. E, Mah, T, Ferrell, R. E, et al. Candidate gene analysis suggests a role for fatty acid biosynthesis and regulation of the complement system in the etiology of age-related maculopathy. *Hum.Mol.Genet.* (2005). , 14, 1991-2002.

[113] Klaver, C. C, Kliffen, M, Van Duijn, C. M, Hofman, A, Cruts, M, Grobbee, D. E, et al. Genetic association of apolipoprotein E with age-related macular degeneration. *Am.J.Hum.Genet.* (1998). , 63, 200-6.

[114] Souied, E. H, Benlian, P, Amouyel, P, Feingold, J, Lagarde, J. P, Munnich, A, et al. The epsilon4 allele of the apolipoprotein E gene as a potential protective factor for exudative age-related macular degeneration. *Am J Ophthalmol* (1998). , 125, 353-9.

[115] Schmidt, S, Klaver, C, Saunders, A, & Postel, E. De La PM, Agarwal A et al. A pooled case-control study of the apolipoprotein E (APOE) gene in age-related maculopathy. *Ophthalmic Genet.* (2002). , 23, 209-23.

[116] Baird, P. N, Guida, E, Chu, D. T, Vu, H. T, & Guymer, R. H. The epsilon2 and epsilon4 alleles of the apolipoprotein gene are associated with age-related macular degeneration. *Invest Ophthalmol.Vis.Sci.* (2004). , 45, 1311-5.

[117] Edwards, A. O, & Ritter, R. III, Abel KJ, Manning A, Panhuysen C, Farrer LA. Complement factor H polymorphism and age-related macular degeneration. *Science* (2005). , 308, 421-4.

[118] Haines, J. L, Hauser, M. A, Schmidt, S, Scott, W. K, Olson, L. M, Gallins, P, et al. Complement factor H variant increases the risk of age-related macular degeneration. *Science* (2005). , 308, 419-21.

[119] Klein, R. J, Zeiss, C, Chew, E. Y, Tsai, J. Y, Sackler, R. S, Haynes, C, et al. Complement factor H polymorphism in age-related macular degeneration. *Science* (2005). , 308, 385-9.

[120] Hageman, G. S, Anderson, D. H, Johnson, L. V, Hancox, L. S, Taiber, A. J, Hardisty, L. I, et al. A common haplotype in the complement regulatory gene factor H (HF1/CFH) predisposes individuals to age-related macular degeneration. *Proc.Natl.Acad.Sci.U.S.A* (2005). , 102, 7227-32.

[121] Gold, B, Merriam, J. E, Zernant, J, Hancox, L. S, Taiber, A. J, Gehrs, K, et al. Variation in factor B (BF) and complement component 2 (C2) genes is associated with age-related macular degeneration. *Nat.Genet.* (2006). , 38, 458-62.

[122] Yates, J. R, Sepp, T, Matharu, B. K, Khan, J. C, Thurlby, D. A, Shahid, H, et al. Complement C3 variant and the risk of age-related macular degeneration. *N.Engl.J.Med.* (2007). , 357, 553-61.

[123] Li, M, Atmaca-sonmez, P, Othman, M, Branham, K. E, Khanna, R, Wade, M. S, et al. CFH haplotypes without the Y402H coding variant show strong association with susceptibility to age-related macular degeneration. *Nat.Genet.* (2006). , 38, 1049-54.

[124] Maller, J, George, S, Purcell, S, Fagerness, J, Altshuler, D, Daly, M. J, et al. Common variation in three genes, including a noncoding variant in CFH, strongly influences risk of age-related macular degeneration. *Nat.Genet.* (2006). , 38, 1055-9.

[125] Yang, Z, Camp, N. J, Sun, H, Tong, Z, Gibbs, D, Cameron, D. J, et al. A variant of the HTRA1 gene increases susceptibility to age-related macular degeneration. *Science* (2006). , 314, 992-3.

[126] Fisher, S. A, Rivera, A, Fritsche, L. G, Babadjanova, G, Petrov, S, & Weber, B. H. Assessment of the contribution of CFH and chromosome 10q26 AMD susceptibility loci in a Russian population isolate. *Br.J.Ophthalmol.* (2007). , 91, 576-8.

[127] Jakobsdottir, J, Conley, Y. P, Weeks, D. E, Mah, T. S, Ferrell, R. E, & Gorin, M. B. Susceptibility genes for age-related maculopathy on chromosome 10q26. *Am.J.Hum.Genet.* (2005). , 77, 389-407.

[128] Van Leeuwen, R, Ikram, M. K, Vingerling, J. R, Witteman, J. C, Hofman, A, & De Jong, P. T. Blood pressure, atherosclerosis, and the incidence of age-related maculopathy: the Rotterdam Study. *Invest Ophthalmol Vis.Sci.* (2003). , 44, 3771-7.

[129] Snow, K. K, & Seddon, J. M. Do age-related macular degeneration and cardiovascular disease share common antecedents? *Ophthalmic Epidemiol.* (1999). , 6, 125-43.

[130] Clemons, T. E, Milton, R. C, Klein, R, Seddon, J. M, & Ferris, F. L. III. Risk factors for the incidence of Advanced Age-Related Macular Degeneration in the Age-Related Eye Disease Study (AREDS) AREDS report *Ophthalmology* (2005). , 112(19), 533-9.

[131] Vinding, T, Appleyard, M, Nyboe, J, & Jensen, G. Risk factor analysis for atrophic and exudative age-related macular degeneration. An epidemiological study of 1000 aged individuals. *Acta Ophthalmol. (Copenh)* (1992). , 70, 66-72.

[132] Smith, W, Mitchell, P, Leeder, S. R, & Wang, J. J. Plasma fibrinogen levels, other cardiovascular risk factors, and age-related maculopathy: the Blue Mountains Eye Study. *Arch.Ophthalmol.* (1998). , 116, 583-7.

[133] Klein, R, Clegg, L, Cooper, L. S, Hubbard, L. D, Klein, B. E, King, W. N, et al. Prevalence of age-related maculopathy in the Atherosclerosis Risk in Communities Study. *Arch.Ophthalmol.* (1999). , 117, 1203-10.

[134] Delcourt, C, Diaz, J. L, Ponton-sanchez, A, & Papoz, L. Smoking and age-related macular degeneration. The POLA Study. Pathologies Oculaires Liees a l'Age. *Arch.Ophthalmol.* (1998). , 116, 1031-5.

[135] Klein, R, Klein, B. E, Tomany, S. C, & Cruickshanks, K. J. The association of cardiovascular disease with the long-term incidence of age-related maculopathy: the Beaver Dam Eye Study. *Ophthalmology* (2003). , 110, 1273-80.

[136] Tomany, S. C, Wang, J. J, Van Leeuwen, R, Klein, R, Mitchell, P, Vingerling, J. R, et al. Risk factors for incident age-related macular degeneration: pooled findings from 3 continents. *Ophthalmology* (2004). , 111, 1280-7.

[137] Buch, H, & Vinding, T. la Cour M, Jensen GB, Prause JU, Nielsen NV. Risk factors for age-related maculopathy in a 14-year follow-up study: the Copenhagen City Eye Study. *Acta Ophthalmol.Scand.* (2005). , 83, 409-18.

[138] Xu, L, Li, Y, Zheng, Y, & Jonas, J. B. Associated factors for age related maculopathy in the adult population in China: the Beijing eye study. *Br.J Ophthalmol.* (2006). , 90, 1087-90.

[139] Klein, R, Deng, Y, Klein, B. E, Hyman, L, Seddon, J, Frank, R. N, et al. Cardiovascular disease, its risk factors and treatment, and age-related macular degeneration: Wom-

en's Health Initiative Sight Exam ancillary study. *Am.J Ophthalmol.* (2007). , 143, 473-83.

[140] Duan, Y, Mo, J, Klein, R, Scott, I. U, Lin, H. M, Caulfield, J, et al. Age-related macular degeneration is associated with incident myocardial infarction among elderly Americans. *Ophthalmology* (2007). , 114, 732-7.

[141] Goldberg, J, Flowerdew, G, Smith, E, Brody, J. A, & Tso, M. O. Factors associated with age-related macular degeneration. An analysis of data from the first National Health and Nutrition Examination Survey. *Am J Epidemiol.* (1988). , 128, 700-10.

[142] Sperduto, R. D, & Hiller, R. Systemic hypertension and age-related maculopathy in the Framingham Study. *Arch.Ophthalmol.* (1986). , 104, 216-9.

[143] Hyman, L, Schachat, A. P, He, Q, & Leske, M. C. Hypertension, cardiovascular disease, and age-related macular degeneration. Age-Related Macular Degeneration Risk Factors Study Group. *Arch.Ophthalmol.* (2000). , 118, 351-8.

[144] Mccarty, C. A, Mukesh, B. N, Fu, C. L, Mitchell, P, Wang, J. J, & Taylor, H. R. Risk factors for age-related maculopathy: the Visual Impairment Project. *Arch.Ophthalmol.* (2001). , 119, 1455-62.

[145] Seddon, J. M, Cote, J, Davis, N, & Rosner, B. Progression of age-related macular degeneration: association with body mass index, waist circumference, and waist-hip ratio. *Arch.Ophthalmol* (2003). , 121, 785-92.

[146] Krishnaiah, S, Das, T, Nirmalan, P. K, Nutheti, R, Shamanna, B. R, Rao, G. N, et al. Risk factors for age-related macular degeneration: findings from the Andhra Pradesh eye disease study in South India. *Invest Ophthalmol.Vis.Sci.* (2005). , 46, 4442-9.

[147] Leske, M. C, Wu, S. Y, Hennis, A, Nemesure, B, Yang, L, Hyman, L, et al. Nine-year incidence of age-related macular degeneration in the Barbados Eye Studies. *Ophthalmology* (2006). , 113, 29-35.

[148] Blumenkranz, M. S, Russell, S. R, Robey, M. G, Kott-blumenkranz, R, & Penneys, N. Risk factors in age-related maculopathy complicated by choroidal neovascularization. *Ophthalmology* (1986). , 93, 552-8.

[149] Klein, R, Klein, B. E, & Jensen, S. C. The relation of cardiovascular disease and its risk factors to the 5-year incidence of age-related maculopathy: the Beaver Dam Eye Study. *Ophthalmology* (1997). , 104, 1804-12.

[150] Vingerling, J. R, Dielemans, I, Bots, M. L, Hofman, A, Grobbee, D. E, & De Jong, P. T. Age-related macular degeneration is associated with atherosclerosis. The Rotterdam Study. *Am J Epidemiol.* (1995). , 142, 404-9.

[151] Curcio, C. A, Millican, C. L, Bailey, T, & Kruth, H. S. Accumulation of cholesterol with age in human Bruch's membrane. *Invest Ophthalmol.Vis.Sci.* (2001). , 42, 265-74.

[152] Tan, J. S, Mitchell, P, Smith, W, & Wang, J. J. Cardiovascular risk factors and the long-term incidence of age-related macular degeneration: the Blue Mountains Eye Study. *Ophthalmology* (2007). , 114, 1143-50.

[153] Lip, P. L, Blann, A. D, Hope-ross, M, Gibson, J. M, & Lip, G. Y. Age-related macular degeneration is associated with increased vascular endothelial growth factor, hemorheology and endothelial dysfunction. *Ophthalmology* (2001). , 108, 705-10.

[154] Lawlor, D. A, Smith, G. D, Rumley, A, Lowe, G. D, & Ebrahim, S. Associations of fibrinogen and C-reactive protein with prevalent and incident coronary heart disease are attenuated by adjustment for confounding factors. British Women's Heart and Health Study. *Thromb.Haemost.* (2005). , 93, 955-63.

[155] Tomany, S. C, Wang, J. J, Van Leeuwen, R, Klein, R, Mitchell, P, Vingerling, J. R, et al. Risk factors for incident age-related macular degeneration: pooled findings from 3 continents. *Ophthalmology* (2004). , 111, 1280-7.

[156] Klein, B. E, Klein, R, & Lee, K. E. Diabetes, cardiovascular disease, selected cardiovascular disease risk factors, and the 5-year incidence of age-related cataract and progression of lens opacities: the Beaver Dam Eye Study. *Am J Ophthalmol* (1998). , 126, 782-90.

[157] Klein, R, Klein, B. E, & Franke, T. The relationship of cardiovascular disease and its risk factors to age-related maculopathy. The Beaver Dam Eye Study. *Ophthalmology* (1993). , 100, 406-14.

[158] Seddon, J. M, Gensler, G, Milton, R. C, Klein, M. L, & Rifai, N. Association between C-reactive protein and age-related macular degeneration. *JAMA* (2004). , 291, 704-10.

[159] Wong, T. Y, Klein, R, Sun, C, Mitchell, P, Couper, D. J, Lai, H, et al. Age-related macular degeneration and risk for stroke. *Ann.Intern.Med.* (2006). , 145, 98-106.

[160] Seddon, J. M, Cote, J, Davis, N, & Rosner, B. Progression of age-related macular degeneration: association with body mass index, waist circumference, and waist-hip ratio. *Arch.Ophthalmol.* (2003). , 121, 785-92.

[161] Schaumberg, D. A, Christen, W. G, Hankinson, S. E, & Glynn, R. J. Body mass index and the incidence of visually significant age-related maculopathy in men. *Arch.Ophthalmol.* (2001). , 119, 1259-65.

[162] Hirvela, H, Luukinen, H, Laara, E, Sc, L, & Laatikainen, L. Risk factors of age-related maculopathy in a population 70 years of age or older. *Ophthalmology* (1996). , 103, 871-7.

[163] Klein, R, Klein, B. E, & Moss, S. E. Diabetes, hyperglycemia, and age-related maculopathy. The Beaver Dam Eye Study. *Ophthalmology* (1992). , 99, 1527-34.

[164] Mitchell, P, & Wang, J. J. Diabetes, fasting blood glucose and age-related maculopathy: The Blue Mountains Eye Study. *Aust.N.Z.J Ophthalmol.* (1999). , 27, 197-9.

[165] Wang, J. J, Klein, R, Smith, W, Klein, B. E, Tomany, S, & Mitchell, P. Cataract surgery and the 5-year incidence of late-stage age-related maculopathy: pooled findings from the Beaver Dam and Blue Mountains eye studies. *Ophthalmology* (2003). , 110, 1960-7.

[166] Fraser-bell, S, Wu, J, Klein, R, Azen, S. P, Hooper, C, Foong, A. W, et al. Cardiovascular risk factors and age-related macular degeneration: the Los Angeles Latino Eye Study. *Am.J.Ophthalmol.* (2008). , 145, 308-16.

[167] Delcourt, C, Michel, F, Colvez, A, Lacroux, A, Delage, M, & Vernet, M. H. Associations of cardiovascular disease and its risk factors with age-related macular degeneration: the POLA study. *Ophthalmic Epidemiol* (2001). , 8, 237-49.

[168] Klein, R, Klein, B. E, Tomany, S. C, & Cruickshanks, K. J. Association of emphysema, gout, and inflammatory markers with long-term incidence of age-related maculopathy. *Arch.Ophthalmol* (2003). , 121, 674-8.

[169] Le, F, Laumet, I, Richard, G, Fievet, F, Berr, N, & Rouaud, C. O et al. Association study of the CFH Y402H polymorphism with Alzheimer's disease. *Neurobiol.Aging* (2010). , 31, 165-6.

[170] Klein, R, Klein, B. E, Linton, K. L, & Demets, D. L. The Beaver Dam Eye Study: the relation of age-related maculopathy to smoking. *Am J Epidemiol.* (1993). , 137, 190-200.

[171] Vingerling, J. R, Hofman, A, Grobbee, D. E, & De Jong, P. T. Age-related macular degeneration and smoking. The Rotterdam Study. *Arch.Ophthalmol.* (1996). , 114, 1193-6.

[172] Christen, W. G, Glynn, R. J, Manson, J. E, Ajani, U. A, & Buring, J. E. A prospective study of cigarette smoking and risk of age-related macular degeneration in men. *JAMA* (1996). , 276, 1147-51.

[173] Seddon, J. M, Willett, W. C, Speizer, F. E, & Hankinson, S. E. A prospective study of cigarette smoking and age-related macular degeneration in women. *JAMA* (1996). , 276, 1141-6.

[174] Smith, W, Mitchell, P, & Leeder, S. R. Smoking and age-related maculopathy. The Blue Mountains Eye Study. *Arch.Ophthalmol.* (1996). , 114, 1518-23.

[175] Maltzman, B. A, Mulvihill, M. N, & Greenbaum, A. Senile macular degeneration and risk factors: a case-control study. *Ann.Ophthalmol.* (1979). , 11, 1197-201.

[176] West, S. K, Rosenthal, F. S, Bressler, N. M, Bressler, S. B, Munoz, B, Fine, S. L, et al. Exposure to sunlight and other risk factors for age-related macular degeneration. *Arch.Ophthalmol.* (1989). , 107, 875-9.

[177] Khan, J. C, Thurlby, D. A, Shahid, H, Clayton, D. G, Yates, J. R, Bradley, M, et al. Smoking and age related macular degeneration: the number of pack years of cigarette smoking is a major determinant of risk for both geographic atrophy and choroidal neovascularisation. *Br.J.Ophthalmol.* (2006). , 90, 75-80.

[178] Coleman, A. L, Seitzman, R. L, Cummings, S. R, Yu, F, Cauley, J. A, Ensrud, K. E, et al. The association of smoking and alcohol use with age-related macular degenera-

tion in the oldest old: the Study of Osteoporotic Fractures. *Am.J.Ophthalmol.* (2010). , 149, 160-9.

[179] Chakravarthy, U, Augood, C, Bentham, G. C, De Jong, P. T, Rahu, M, Seland, J, et al. Cigarette smoking and age-related macular degeneration in the EUREYE Study. *Ophthalmology* (2007). , 114, 1157-63.

[180] Aoki, K, Ito, Y, Sasaki, R, Ohtani, M, Hamajima, N, & Asano, A. Smoking, alcohol drinking and serum carotenoids levels. *Jpn.J Cancer Res.* (1987). , 78, 1049-56.

[181] Hammond, B. R. Jr., Wooten BR, Snodderly DM. Cigarette smoking and retinal carotenoids: implications for age-related macular degeneration. *Vision Res.* (1996). , 36, 3003-9.

[182] Kew, R. R, Ghebrehiwet, B, & Janoff, A. Cigarette smoke can activate the alternative pathway of complement in vitro by modifying the third component of complement. *J Clin.Invest* (1985). , 75, 1000-7.

[183] Sastry, B. V, & Hemontolor, M. E. Influence of nicotine and cotinine on retinal phospholipase A2 and its significance to macular function. *J Ocul.Pharmacol.Ther.* (1998). , 14, 447-58.

[184] Espinosa-heidmann, D. G, Suner, I. J, Catanuto, P, Hernandez, E. P, Marin-castano, M. E, & Cousins, S. W. Cigarette smoke-related oxidants and the development of sub-RPE deposits in an experimental animal model of dry AMD. *Invest Ophthalmol.Vis.Sci.* (2006). , 47, 729-37.

[185] Wassell, J, Davies, S, Bardsley, W, & Boulton, M. The photoreactivity of the retinal age pigment lipofuscin. *J Biol.Chem.* (1999). , 274, 23828-32.

[186] Brunk, U. T, Wihlmark, U, Wrigstad, A, Roberg, K, & Nilsson, S. E. Accumulation of lipofuscin within retinal pigment epithelial cells results in enhanced sensitivity to photo-oxidation. *Gerontology* (1995). Suppl , 2, 201-12.

[187] Fekrat, S, & Bressler, S. B. Are antioxidants or other supplements protective for age-related macular degeneration? *Curr.Opin.Ophthalmol.* (1996). , 7, 65-72.

[188] Taylor, H. R, West, S, Munoz, B, Rosenthal, F. S, Bressler, S. B, & Bressler, N. M. The long-term effects of visible light on the eye. *Arch.Ophthalmol.* (1992). , 110, 99-104.

[189] Cruickshanks, K. J, Klein, R, & Klein, B. E. Sunlight and age-related macular degeneration. The Beaver Dam Eye Study. *Arch.Ophthalmol.* (1993). , 111, 514-8.

[190] Tso, M. O, Woodford, B. J, & Lam, K. W. Distribution of ascorbate in normal primate retina and after photic injury: a biochemical, morphological correlated study. *Curr.Eye Res.* (1984). , 3, 181-91.

[191] Organisciak, D. T, Jiang, Y. L, Wang, H. M, & Bicknell, I. The protective effect of ascorbic acid in retinal light damage of rats exposed to intermittent light. *Invest Ophthalmol Vis.Sci.* (1990). , 31, 1195-202.

[192] Hayes, K. C. Pathophysiology of vitamin E deficiency in monkeys. *Am.J.Clin.Nutr.* (1974)., 27, 1130-40.

[193] Leure-dupree, A. E, & Mcclain, C. J. The effect of severe zinc deficiency on the morphology of the rat retinal pigment epithelium. *Invest Ophthalmol.Vis.Sci.* (1982)., 23, 425-34.

[194] Hollis, A. L, Butcher, W. I, Davis, H, Henderson, R. A, & Stone, W. L. Structural alterations in retinal tissues from rats deficient in vitamin E and selenium and treated with hyperbaric oxygen. *Exp.Eye Res.* (1992)., 54, 671-84.

[195] Antioxidant status and neovascular age-related macular degenerationEye Disease Case-Control Study Group. *Arch Ophthalmol* (1993)., 111, 104-9.

[196] Seddon, J. M, Ajani, U. A, Sperduto, R. D, Hiller, R, Blair, N, Burton, T. C, et al. Dietary carotenoids, vitamins A, C, and E, and advanced age-related macular degeneration. Eye Disease Case-Control Study Group. *JAMA* (1994)., 272, 1413-20.

[197] Mares-perlman, J. A, Klein, R, Klein, B. E, Greger, J. L, Brady, W. E, Palta, M, et al. Association of zinc and antioxidant nutrients with age-related maculopathy. *Arch Ophthalmol* (1996)., 114, 991-7.

[198] Mares-perlman, J. A, Fisher, A. I, Klein, R, Palta, M, Block, G, Millen, A. E, et al. Lutein and zeaxanthin in the diet and serum and their relation to age-related maculopathy in the third national health and nutrition examination survey. *Am J Epidemiol.* (2001)., 153, 424-32.

[199] Randomized, A. placebo-controlled, clinical trial of high-dose supplementation with vitamins C and E, beta carotene, and zinc for age-related macular degeneration and vision loss: AREDS report *Arch Ophthalmol* (2001)., 119(8), 1417-36.

[200] The Age-Related Eye Disease Study 2 (AREDS2): A Multi-CenterRandomized Trial of lutein, Zeaxanthin, and Omega-3 Long-Chain Polyunsaturated Fatty Acids (Docosahexaenoic Acid [DHA] and Eicosapentaenoic Acid [EPA]) in Age-Related Macular Degeneration. (2008). http://clinicalstudies.info.nih.gov/cgi/wais/bold032001.pl?A_EI-0025.html@lutein.

[201] Cho, E, Hung, S, Willett, W. C, Spiegelman, D, Rimm, E. B, Seddon, J. M, et al. Prospective study of dietary fat and the risk of age-related macular degeneration. *Am.J Clin.Nutr.* (2001)., 73, 209-18.

[202] Mares-perlman, J. A, Brady, W. E, & Klein, R. VandenLangenberg GM, Klein BE, Palta M. Dietary fat and age-related maculopathy. *Arch.Ophthalmol.* (1995)., 113, 743-8.

[203] Seddon, J. M, Cote, J, & Rosner, B. Progression of age-related macular degeneration: association with dietary fat, transunsaturated fat, nuts, and fish intake. *Arch.Ophthalmol.* (2003)., 121, 1728-37.

[204] Seddon, J. M, Rosner, B, Sperduto, R. D, Yannuzzi, L, Haller, J. A, Blair, N. P, et al. Dietary fat and risk for advanced age-related macular degeneration. *Arch Ophthalmol* (2001). , 119, 1191-9.

[205] Chua, B, Flood, V, Rochtchina, E, Wang, J. J, Smith, W, & Mitchell, P. Dietary fatty acids and the 5-year incidence of age-related maculopathy. *Arch.Ophthalmol.* (2006). , 124, 981-6.

[206] Hodge, W. G, Schachter, H. M, Barnes, D, Pan, Y, Lowcock, E. C, Zhang, L, et al. Efficacy of omega-3 fatty acids in preventing age-related macular degeneration: a systematic review. *Ophthalmology* (2006). , 113, 1165-72.

[207] Hodge, W. G, Barnes, D, Schachter, H. M, Pan, Y. I, Lowcock, E. C, Zhang, L, et al. Evidence for the effect of omega-3 fatty acids on progression of age-related macular degeneration: a systematic review. *Retina* (2007). , 27, 216-21.

[208] Bora, P. S, Kaliappan, S, Xu, Q, Kumar, S, Wang, Y, Kaplan, H. J, et al. Alcohol linked to enhanced angiogenesis in rat model of choroidal neovascularization. *FEBS J* (2006). , 273, 1403-14.

[209] Miyazaki, M, Nakamura, H, Kubo, M, Kiyohara, Y, Oshima, Y, Ishibashi, T, et al. Risk factors for age related maculopathy in a Japanese population: the Hisayama study. *Br.J Ophthalmol.* (2003). , 87, 469-72.

[210] Ajani, U. A, Christen, W. G, Manson, J. E, Glynn, R. J, Schaumberg, D, Buring, J. E, et al. A prospective study of alcohol consumption and the risk of age-related macular degeneration. *Ann.Epidemiol* (1999). , 9, 172-7.

[211] Boekhoorn, S. S, Vingerling, J. R, Hofman, A, & De Jong, P. T. Alcohol consumption and risk of aging macula disorder in a general population: the Rotterdam Study. *Arch.Ophthalmol.* (2008). , 126, 834-9.

[212] Moss, S. E, Klein, R, Klein, B. E, Jensen, S. C, & Meuer, S. M. Alcohol consumption and the 5-year incidence of age-related maculopathy: the Beaver Dam eye study. *Ophthalmology* (1998). , 105, 789-94.

[213] Cho, E, Hankinson, S. E, Willett, W. C, Stampfer, M. J, Spiegelman, D, Speizer, F. E, et al. Prospective study of alcohol consumption and the risk of age-related macular degeneration. *Arch.Ophthalmol.* (2000). , 118, 681-8.

[214] Klein, R, Klein, B. E, Tomany, S. C, & Moss, S. E. Ten-year incidence of age-related maculopathy and smoking and drinking: the Beaver Dam Eye Study. *Am J Epidemiol.* (2002). , 156, 589-98.

[215] Deangelis, M. M, Lane, A. M, Shah, C. P, Ott, J, Dryja, T. P, & Miller, J. W. Extremely discordant sib-pair study design to determine risk factors for neovascular age-related macular degeneration. *Arch.Ophthalmol.* (2004). , 122, 575-80.

[216] Ritter, L. L, Klein, R, Klein, B. E, Mares-perlman, J. A, & Jensen, S. C. Alcohol use and age-related maculopathy in the Beaver Dam Eye Study. *Am.J Ophthalmol.* (1995). , 120, 190-6.

[217] Knudtson, M. D, Klein, R, & Klein, B. E. Alcohol consumption and the 15-year cumulative incidence of age-related macular degeneration. *Am.J Ophthalmol.* (2007). , 143, 1026-9.

[218] Arnarsson, A, Sverrisson, T, Stefansson, E, Sigurdsson, H, Sasaki, H, Sasaki, K, et al. Risk factors for five-year incident age-related macular degeneration: the Reykjavik Eye Study. *Am.J Ophthalmol.* (2006). , 142, 419-28.

[219] Chong, E. W, Kreis, A. J, Wong, T. Y, Simpson, J. A, & Guymer, R. H. Alcohol consumption and the risk of age-related macular degeneration: a systematic review and meta-analysis. *Am.J Ophthalmol.* (2008). , 145, 707-15.

Chapter 2

Cigarette Smoking and Hypertension Two Risk Factors for Age-Related Macular Degeneration

Maria E. Marin-Castaño

Additional information is available at the end of the chapter

http://dx.doi.org/10.5772/53958

1. Introduction

1.1. Age-related macular degeneration

Age-related macular degeneration (AMD) is a progressive retinal degeneration that is untreatable in up to 90% of patients and is the leading cause of blindness in the elderly worldwide [1]. Although much effort is invested in understanding this condition, there is neither a cure nor a way to prevent it, and treatment options are very limited. AMD affects 30% of people age 70 or older, and 60 million people worldwide are affected. Over 10 million people are affected in the United States and it is estimated that more than 300,000 new cases are diagnosed annually [2-4]. Since persons over 60 represent the fastest growing segment of the population, AMD will remain a significant public health problem for the foreseeable future [5,6].

AMD is a multifactorial disease with age, systemic health, genetic and environmental risk factors influencing disease progression [7, 8]. The most important pathogenic factors leading up to AMD include oxidative stress, inflammation, and local production of angiogenic factors [9]. A substantial body of literature suggests a role for oxidant injury to the RPE and local inflammation as putative mechanisms in the pathogenesis of AMD [10-12]. However, to date, little is known about the molecular signal(s) linking oxidation to inflammation in this late-onset disease.

In AMD loss or dysfunction of retinal photoreceptors is the ultimate cause of vision loss. However, the initial pathogenic target of AMD is the retinal pigment epithelium (RPE), Brusch's membrane (BrM), and choriochapillaris [13,14]. Clinical manifestations of AMD may present in early or a late form [15]. In early AMD (commonly known as dry degeneration) (Fig. 1B), variuos lipic-derived and protein-rich extracellular deposits, known as drusen, accumulate under the RPE (Fig. 2) [14-16]. Ultimately, early AMD can progress to the late form of the disease; geographic atrophy (commonly known as advanced dry AMD) (Fig. 1C) or neovascular AMD (commonly known as wet or exudative AMD) (Fig. 1D). Geographic atrophy is characterized by death of RPE and photoreceptors (Fig. 1C) [14,15].

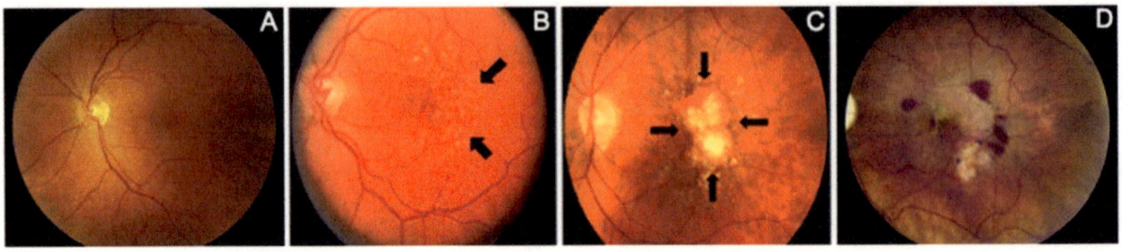

Figure 1. Fundus Photographs in health, early age-related macular degeneration (AMD), late forms of atrophic AMD and neovascular AMD. The ocular fundus of a healthy eye, showing normal pigmentation and retinal blood vessels (A). Drusen (thick arrows), seen as multiple discrete round yellow sub-retinal pigment epithelium (RPE) deposits, are the first sign of early AMD (B). Atrophic AMD (C) is characterized by a window defect (thin arrows) with loss of RPE and overlying photoreceptors. Neovascular AMD (D) is characterized by choroidal neovascularization (CNV), which is prone to fluid exudation, hemorrhage, and fibrosis. The late-stage dry form of AMD, known as geographic atrophy. Note large regions of depigmentation, especially in the macula, which is at the center of the image.(C) In wet AMD, leaky blood vessels from the choroid invade the overlying retina.

Neovascular AMD is characterized by the growth of new abnormal blood vessels, with leaky walls, under the RPE from the subjacent choroid, resulting in choroidal neovascularization (CNV) and subsequent dysfunction or death of the overlying neurosensory retina [14,15]. Neovascular AMD progresses much more rapidly than early AMD and leads to a greater loss of central vision. What both forms have in common, however, is pathology at the RPE/choroid interface, which includes a thickening of BrM, due to the deposition of extracellular material between the RPE and BrM (sub-RPE deposits and drusen) (Fig. 2). This review will focus on the pathobiology of the early AMD by exploring the role of cigarette smoking and hypertension in the onset and development of the disease.

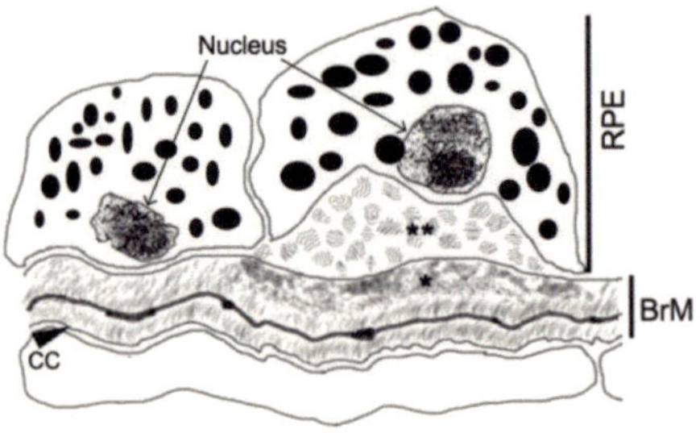

Figure 2. Schematic image of the RPE-Bruch's membrane-choriocapillaris interface in AMD. Basal laminar deposits (BLD; **) appear between the RPE cell and the RPE basement membrane, while basal linear deposits (BlinD; *) localize at the inner collagenous layer beneath the RPE basement membrane. Arrowhead indicates endothelial cell basement membrane.

2. The outer retina and choroid

As mentioned above, the pathology at the RPE/choroid interface, which includes deposition of extracellular material between the RPE and BrM, is what both AMD forms have in common. BrM undergoes several biochemical and anatomical changes with aging, including collagenous thickening, calcification, and lipid infiltration, in the absence of apparent retinal dysfunction [17,18]. The accumulation of specific deposits under the RPE is the hallmark histopathological feature of eyes with early AMD, when visual function is still not irreversibly impaired [14,19].

The RPE is a monolayer of hexagonally arranged, highly pigmented cells, located between the neural retina and the choroid, and forming part of the blood-retina barrier (Fig. 3). Its many functions include; the absorption of light that did not get captured by the photoreceptor outer segment pigments; epithelial transport of molecules (nutrients, ions, water, and metabolites) between the subretinal space and the choroidal blood supply; spatial ion buffering; re-isomerization of the chromophore 11-cis-retinal from all-trans retinal; the daily removal of photoreceptor outer segments by phagocytosis; the secretion of molecules such as growth factors, proteases, and others that control the stability of the photoreceptor cells, BrM and the choroid; and finally, the modulation of the immune response, since the RPE participates in control of the immune privilege in the healthy eye or the mounting of an immune response in the diseased eye [20]. Abnormalities in any of these processes might participate in RPE cell pathology.

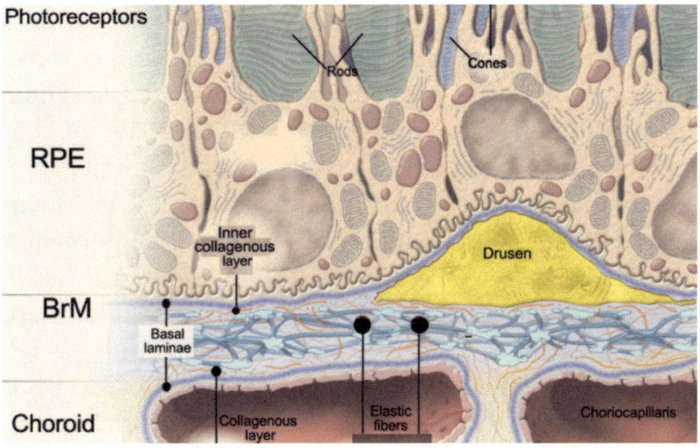

Figure 3. Schematic image of the photoreceptors-RPE-Bruch's membrane-choriocapillaris interface and drusen in AMD.

BrM occupies a crucial interface between the RPE and choroid and contains the basement membrane of both the RPE and choroid (Fig. 3). BrM is traditionally considered to be a five-layered stratified extracellular matrix that provides structural support to the overlying RPE and retina [6,18,21]. BrM also provides a semipermeable filtration barrier through which major metabolic exchange takes place between the RPE and the choriocapillaris. In the center of BrM is the elastic fiber layer (Fig. 3) sandwiched between the inner and outer collagenous layers. Finally, two basal laminas define the innermost and outermost layers. The innermost layer is the basal lamina of the RPE; the outermost layer is formed by the basement membrane of the endothelial cells that comprise the choriocapillaris [6,18,21]. The collagen layers contain striated collagen fibers mainly type I, III, and V [6,18]. Type I confers tensile strength to the tissue, type III is normally present in tissues with elastic properties, and type V acts to anchor basement membranes to stromal matrixes [17,18]. The interfiber matrix of BrM is comprised largely of glycosaminoglycans such as heparan sulfate (25%) and chondroitin/dermatan sulfate (75%). These provide an electrolytic barrier to diffusion and serve important regulatory roles by binding extracellular proteins and growth factors that are vital for cellular processes such as adhesion, migration, and differentiation [17,22,23].

The basement membrane of both the choriocapillaris and RPE are comprised of mostly type IV collagen [17,18]. The basement membranes additionally contain laminin, heparan sulfate, proteoglycans, and fibronectin. The outermost basal lamina also incorporates type VI collagen, which is associated with the choriocapillaris [17,18]. It has been suggested that this collagen may act to anchor fenestrated capillaries to the underlying choroid.

3. Subretinal deposit formation and progression: Pathogenic mechanisms

The accumulation of specific deposits under the RPE is a very prominent histopathologic feature of eyes with AMD [24-27]. Sub-RPE deposits were first described nearly 160 years ago and were generically termed "drusen" when observed by ophthalmologists upon clinical examination of the retina [28]. Histopathological examination defines three main types of sub-RPE deposits on the basis of thickness, content, and locationt: a) basal laminar deposits (BLD), b) basal linear deposits (BLinD), and c) nodular drusen [14,29,30]. BLD and BLinD are both diffuse deposits that accumulate on opposite sides of the basal lamina of the RPE (Fig. 2); therefore, the RPE basement membrane is the crucial dividing line that demarcates the location of BLD from BLinD [14]. BLD is seen as amorphous material of intermediate electron density between the plasma membrane and the basement membrane of the RPE, often containing wide-spaced collagen, patches of electron-dense fibrillar or granular material, and occasionally, membranous debris [31]. They are distributed throughout the retina, including the periphery as well as the macula, underlying not only cones but rods as well. BLinD are diffuse, amorphous accumulations within the inner collagenous zone of BrM, external to RPE basement membrane (Fig. 2), with similar content variations [14]. BLinD are characterized by coated and non-coated vesicles as well as some membranous and empty profiles [14]. Biochemically, deposits contain phospholipids, triglycerides, cholesterol, cholesterol esters, unsaturated fatty acids, peroxidized lipids, and apolipoproteins [24-26].

Nodular drusen are discrete, dome-shaped deposits within the inner collagenous zone of BrM (i.e., external to the RPE basal lamina), which are often contiguous with BLinD, and can be difficult to distinguish from BLinD without electron microscopy [5]. Nodular drusen may also specifically contain vitronectin, immunoglobulins, amyloid, complement, and proteins associated with RPE cell function [32] as well as other poorly characterized components [24-27]. Further, low-grade monocyte infiltration within the choriocapillaris is often present underlying areas of deposits [25,27,33].

Clinically, deposits of AMD are classified on fundoscopic features of morphology and size [24]. Although multiple classifications exist, most clinicians use size to classify drusen: small or "hard" (<63 μm) and soft, intermediate (>63 to <125 μm) and large (>125 μm) drusen [24]. When hard or soft drusen coalesce to the point of losing their boundaries they are then classified as "diffuse." Although diagnosis of AMD is typically made when intermediate or large drusen are present, the diagnosis can be also be made in the absence of drusen based on the presence of pigmentary changes indicative of RPE degeneration [3,29,30]. The specific contribution of drusen to AMD complications and progression are not well characterized, but the presence of macular drusen is considered a strong risk factor for the development of both forms of late AMD, geographic atrophy and neovascular AMD [3,34,35]. In general, eyes with clinical AMD have been found to express all three deposit subtypes [14,25,36]. Furthermore, histological, immunohistochemical, and ultrastructural studies of surgically-excised choroidal neovascular (CNV) membranes have shown that the cellular and extracellular constituents of CNV are the same regardless of the underlying disease, with the exception of the amount of BLD and the presence of BLinD, which is virtually exclusively found in CNV specimens from patients with AMD [29,37].

The cellular and molecular events involved in drusen formation have not been fully elucidated. Lack of scientific consensus exists regarding the origin of drusen, but at least five different paradigms are currently proposed to explain deposit formation in AMD; a) genetic hypothesis, b) lysosomal failure/lipofuscin hypothesis, c) choroidal hypoperfusion hypothesis, d) barrier hypothesis, and e) RPE injury hypothesis. Because our research is based on the RPE injury hypothesis, in this section this theory is reviewed in light of the more recent finding.

There are a number of direct and/or indirect lines of evidence supporting a role for the RPE in drusen biogenesis. According to traditional models of drusen formation, any cellular material residing within drusen is predicted to be of RPE origin. Indeed, RPE-derived basal laminae, organelles and cellular fragments, and even entire cells can be detected in early "drusen". Some authors have described the appearance of RPE "debris" blebbing into drusen or pre-drusen sites [38]. RPE constituents, such as basal laminae, as well as lipofuscin and melanin granules, are observed within early drusen, where they likely contribute to drusen volume and formation.

The theory that drusen were derived from damaged RPE was originally postulated by Donders, who first described drusen in a post-mortem eye, believed that drusen were derived from RPE nuclei, based on the supposition that the latter are relatively resistant to degradation [39]. Donders' theory was later modified by De Vicentis (1887) who proposed that degenerative change in the RPE cytoplasm, rather than in the nucleus, was the precipitating event. On the other hand, Muller (1856) proposed that drusen result from aberrant secretion of basement membrane components by the aged RPE [40].With the advent of electron microscopy, the substructural features of drusen were revealed, and new variants of the earlier theories were advanced. Some investigators have concluded, that drusen are formed when the RPE expels portions of its basal cytoplasm into BrM [38], possibly as a mechanism for removing damaged cytosol [41] or as a byproduct of phagocytic degradation [19]. Others have postulated that drusen are formed by autolysis of the RPE, due to aberrant lysosomal enzyme activity [42], although enzyme histochemical studies failed to demonstrate the presence of lysosomal enzymes in drusen [43]. Additional mechanisms for drusen formation, including lipoidal degeneration of the RPE, have been proposed [44,45].

In the modern version, the RPE injury hypothesis proposes that deposit formation is secondary to chronic, repetitive but nonlethal RPE injury [46, 47]. Two separate phenomena must be distinguished: the injury stimulus and the cellular response. The most widely implicated injury stimuli are various oxidants, especially those induced by RPE exposure to visible light or those derived from endogenous metabolism [48,49]. More recently, inflammatory-derived injury stimuli have also become implicated, including oxidants, complement, immune complexes and factors produced by macrophages or monocyte [50-52]. Inflammatory cells might be responsible for drusen progression into CNV by secretion of growth factors and cytokines that will damage the choriocapillaris and stimulate the invasion of neovessels into the subretinal space [37,51,52].

Irrespective of the injury, this model proposes that all stimuli result in a final common pathway of cellular responses that cause the actual deposits. Cellular responses that can lead to deposit formation include RPE cell membrane blebbing and dysregulation of extracellular matrix (ECM) production and breakdown. Accumulation of sub-RPE blebbed material in the setting of imbalanced breakdown and resynthesis of basement membrane and BrM ECM is proposed to produce the various deposits of AMD. Repetitive injury ultimately can kill RPE, leading to late dry AMD [6].

4. Hypothetical model for dry AMD and its progression to wet AMD

Our research is based on the RPE injury hypothesis (Fig. 4). Oxidative injury-mediated non lethal RPE membrane blebbing, dysregulation of ECM turnover, inflammation, and angiogenesis appear to be key cellular processes that play a central role in the formation and progression of sub-RPE deposits. We postulate that the pathogenesis and progression of dry AMD is characterized by the following stages: (A) Initial RPE oxidant injury causes extrusion of cell membrane "blebs," together with decreased activity of matrix metalloproteinases (MMPs), promoting bleb accumulation under the RPE as BLD. Numerous endogenous or exogenous oxidants can induce blebbing; (B) RPE cells are subsequently stimulated to increase synthesis of MMPs and other molecules responsible for extracellular matrix turnover (i.e., producing decreased laminin and collagen), affecting both RPE basement membrane and BrM [46,53,54]. This process leads to progression of BLD into BLinD and drusen by admixture of blebs into BrM, followed by the formation of new basement membrane under the RPE to trap these deposits within BrM [55,56]. We postulate that various hormones and other plasma-derived molecules related to systemic health cofactors are implicated in this stage [57-60]. (C) Altered macrophages recruitment to sites of RPE injury and deposit formation. Macrophage

http://dx.doi.org/10.5772/53958

recruitment may be beneficial or harmful depending upon their activation status at the time of recruitment [50,61]. Nonactivated or scavenging macrophages may remove deposits without further injury. Activated or reparative macrophages, through the release of inflammatory mediators, growth factors, or other substances, may promote complications and progression to the late forms of the disease [37,50,62,37]. As discussed below, the effect of cigarette smoking and Ang II in the mentioned stages will be reviewed in depth.

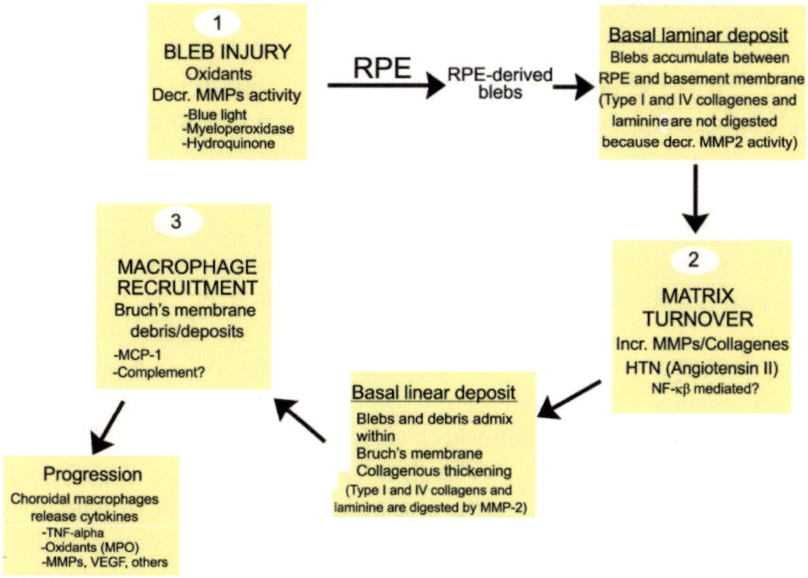

Figure 4. Schematic drawing of the early stages of age-related macular degeneration (AMD). First stage: Oxidant injury at the retinal pigment epithelium (RPE) causes bleb formation and decreased matrix metalloproteinases (MMPs). Blebs than accumulate between the RPE and the basement membrane as basal laminar deposits (BLDs). Second stage: Increased matrix turnover characterized by increased MMPs and decreased collagens. BLDs progress into basal linear deposits (BLinDs) and drusen and are located within the inner collagenous layer of Bruchs membrane. Third stage: Macrophages recruited to the site of injury by chemotactic factors are responsible for release of cytokines, angiogenic factors, and oxidants that perpetuate RPE injury and lead to late stages of AMD. Abbreviations: MPO = myeloperoxidase; NF-κB = nuclear factor kappa-light-chain-enhancer of activated B cells; TNF-α: tumor necrosis factor-alpha; MCP-1: monocyte chemotactic protein-1; VEGF: vascular endothelial growth factor.

5. Smoking and age-related macular degeneration

It has been postulated that environmental oxidants are frequently implicated in RPE injury and may contribute to deposit formation. Cigarette smoking is the strongest environmental risk factor for all forms of AMD, even in people exposed to passive smoking [63-66]. People who have smoked at least 100 cigarettes (lifetime) have approximately triple risk of developing AMD compared to individuals who have never smoked. Current smokers and heavy smokers have even higher AMD risk.

Cigarette smoke is comprised of a gas and tar phase. Each phase contains both inorganic and organic free radicals, including ROS, epoxides, peroxides, NO, nitrogen dioxide, peroxynitrite, peroxynitrates and various other free radicals [67]. Moreover, cigarette smoke contains a high concentration of potent oxidants such as acrolein [68-70], dioxin [71], Benzo(a)Pyrene [72], cadmium, [73-75] quinones, nicotine, and NO [76-79]. Many of them demonstrated to be toxic to ocular tissue affecting the eye through oxidative damage and abnormal vascularization. Although the pathogenesis of AMD and the mechanism of action of smoking on the eye are not fully understood [80], the risk of developing AMD is likely to involve more than one mechanism.

Smoking habit appears to be related to the long-term incidence and progression of AMD [81]. Plausible biological mechanisms such as direct oxidation, depletion of antioxidant protection (e.g. decreases plasma vitamin C and carotenoids), immune system activation, atherosclerotic vascular changes, induction of hypoxia and alteration of choroidal blood flow [82,83], support the involvement of smoking in the etiology of AMD [84]. Interestingly, the Age-related Eye Disease Study (AREDS) [85] found that reduction in plasma glutathione and cysteine oxidation correlated with benefit from anti-oxidant treatment for intermediate AMD [86]. Collectively, these studies, along with the studies on cigarette smoking, implicate oxidative stress as a mechanism of AMD. Genetic variations such as a susceptibility locus in or near the hypothetical LOC387715 gene were associated with AMD [87,88]. It has been reported that this locus encodes a mitochondrial protein, raising suspicion for a role of the oxidative defense response in this disease. This locus is associated with smoking, and the combination of the LOC387715 polymorphism and smoking confers a higher risk for AMD than either factor alone [89,90]. Moreover, chemical in cigarette smoke modifies oxidatively docosohexanoic acid (DHA), the most abundant fatty acid in photoreceptor tips, to carboxyethylpyrrole (CEP) [91] and other lipids which have been identified which "tag" oxidatively oxidized damaged photoreceptors in AMD [92]. In the RPE, multiple proteins isolated from lipofuscin are also oxidatively damaged by cigarette smoke compounds including malondialdehyde, 4-hydroxynonenal and advanced glycation end products (AGE) [93,94]. Interestingly, AGEs accumulate in BrM including basal deposits and drusen, and CEP adducts appear in drusen isolated from AMD samples [95,96].The ability to defend against oxidative stress by upregulating the anti-oxidant defense response is likely to be a pivotal event that mediates the initiation and progression of AMD. The molecular damage from oxidative modification illustrated here, suggests that the anti-oxidant response in the macula at some point, becomes unable to neutralize oxidative stress.

In addition to direct oxidative damage to tissue, oxidative free radicals from cigarette smoke can modulate the immune-inflammatory system in part, through enhanced expression of pro-inflammatory genes, as reviewed in Biswas and Rahman (2009) [97]. The discovery of polymorphisms in several complement factors with AMD susceptibility points toward a specific role for complement mediated inflammation in the pathophysiology of AMD [98,99]. AMD has been associated with local inflammatory responses in the RPE/choroid [100]. In previous works, it was demonstrated that the aged RPE/choroid becomes immunologically active [101] due to increased expression of complement components. Smoking also influences the function of the alternative pathway of complement activation [121]. Smoking seems to alter the C3 component of the complement and to reduce the efficacy by which it binds to complement factor H (CFH).

The association between smoke and ApoE has also been investigated. Smokers are known to have higher serum cholesterol and LDL levels, a possible risk factor for AMD development [102]. Impaired cholesterol metabolism in particular ApoE isoforms carriers could be further enhanced among smokers. Moreover, smoking is associated with decreased endothelial NO production, while ApoE-4 genotype has been reported to increase NO synthesis, relative to ApoE2 and ApoE3 [103]. Thus, the presence of the ApoE2 protein in smokers may reduce endothelial NO levels in cell tissues. Given that the normal function of NO in the retina is to neutralize circulating oxidized lipids, its decreased availability may promote oxidative damage to the RPE cells.

As mentioned above, quinones, acrolein, BenzoPyrenes, and cadmium can damage the eye through oxidative processes. It has been demonstrated that hydroquinone the most abundant quinone in cigarette smoke causes oxidative damage, apoptosis, increases lipid peroxidation and mitochondrial superoxide production, and decreases intracellular glutathione in the RPE cells [104]. Acrolein, a product of lipid peroxidation in vivo, is a mitochondrial toxicant in RPE cells, which induces oxidative mitochondrial dysfunction and oxidative damage to proteins and DNA causing loss of cell viability [70-72]. Whereas Benzo(a)Pyrene causes mtDNA damage, alteration in the lysosomal activity, complement activation in the aged RPE, and upregulates expression of complement pathway components such as C3a, C5, C5b-9, and CFH in the RPE/choroid contributing to drusen formation [105,106]. Cadmium (Cd), is another toxic which is concentrated in the body through cigarette smoke. Cd has been demonstrated to be a potent inflammatory, an oxidant agent, and accumulates with aging, effects which are linked to AMD [77, 107]. In vitro studies have revealed Cd as an important potential factor in RPE cell death associated retinal disease [76].

Cigarette smoke also induces angiogenesis promoting CNV and progression to neovascular AMD. Nicotine is one of the major components of the cigarette and has been demonstrated to enhance the generation of radical oxygen species producing oxidative stress [108-110] and promote the generation of pro-inflammatory responses leading to chronic inflammation in smokers [111]. Futhermore, nicotine is responsible for the mitogenesis of endothelial and smooth muscle cells [112] regulating abnormal responses to vascular injury [113] and endothelial functions [114]. We and other previously showed that nicotine by its direct action on nicotinic receptors promoted angiogenesis and increased size and severity of CNV in a mouse model [112, 114]. Moreover, it has been shown that nicotine targets the retinal microvasculature by reducing the apoptotic rate of vascular endothelial cells and inducing the formation of new capillarity, mediated at least in part by release of vascular endothelial growth factor (VEGF) [113], which is one of the key growth factors involved in neovascularization and implicated in the most severe form of AMD [115-118]. Nicotine has also the ability to stimulate the growth of smooth muscle cells after oxidative injury, leading to the development of CNV in the retina. Moreover other cigarette smoke components such as dioxin induce expression and release of VEGF by RPE cells promoting CNV [104, 119].

6. Hypertension and age-related macular degeneration

Even though age is the major determinant for developing AMD, clinical and epidemiologic studies have suggested systemic vascular disease, especially hypertension, as an important risk factor for AMD [3,119] and a correlation between AMD and aging and hypertension [3, 120]. Aging is the risk factor with the greatest correlation with incidence, prevalence and severity of AMD, but the age-related susceptibility factors remain completely unknown [3,120]. However, increased sensitivity to the injurious effects of hypertension and to oxidant-injury are all more severe in the elderly than in the young [121-123]. For exemple, the interaction of Angiotensin II (Ang II) (the most important hormone associated with hypertension) with AT1 receptors, produces ROS, and with advancing age, oxidative alterations accumulate in cellular components, including those in the antioxidative defense systems, due to disrupted redox regulation during aging can influence the gene transcription and signal transduction pathways.

Hypertension is of particular interest among the systemic risk factors, due to its increasing incidence in Western societies. In several cross sectional and case control studies, systemic hypertension was associated with increased prevalence and progression of the severity and incidence of drusen [124] and with the development of wet AMD [125-127]. Interestingly, a recent study provides a strong association between hypertension and the development of wet AMD in the presence of early AMD [128]. Despite of the apparent link between AMD and hypertension, these studies make no mention of the mechanism(s) by which hypertension may induce or contribute to the pathogenesis of dry AMD and its progression from early AMD to CNV.

Traditionally, hypertension is believed to contribute to chronic diseases by at least two distinct mechanisms: hemodynamic injury and humoral factors [129-131]. Hemodynamic injury refers to mechanical damage induced by flow turbulence in large vessels or stretching of capillaries induced by increased blood pressure. Humoral factors refer to cellular activities induced by hormones or growth factors associated with hypertension [129,130] shuch as Ang II, which is upregulated in hypertension, present in the blood of many hypertensive patients and has been demonstrated to activate specific receptors to induce various cellular functions. Ang II as the molecular surrogate for the effects of hypertension in AMD, and its properties will be described below.

The classical view of the renin-angiotensin system (RAS) as a systemic regulator of blood pressure has been extended, and a substantial number of studies have highlighted the importance of local RAS in a variety of extra-renal tissues, including adrenal glands [132], thymus [133] and recently in the eye [134,135]. In the eye, Ang II, and Ang II type 1 and type 2 receptors (AT1R, AT2R) have been found in the retina, particularly in the retinal pigment epithelium (RPE) [59,60,136-139]. Similarly, studies in rat retinal tissues also suggested local synthesis of both renin and angiotensin convertingenzyme (ACE) [140]. Along this line, Milenkovic et al. (2010) demonstrated that the RPE expresses renin and secretes it towards the retinal side. The presence of the most important RAS components in the retina implies a physiological function of RAS within the eye. However, despite the considerable evidence for local RAS in the retina, its exact role and its possible relationship with the systemic RAS remain poorly understood. The fact that AT1R is localized at the basolateral membrane of the RPE, which faces the blood side of the epithelium, suggests that the activity of the systemic RAS is a part of that signaling. Interestingly, it has been shown that modulation of the systemic RAS (e.g. by systemic application of ACE inhibitors) changes neuronal activity within the retina, mainly of bipolar cells and amacrine cells as monitored by electroretinography [139,141,142]. Moreover, modulators of the systemic RAS alter renin expression in the RPE [138] and plasma Ang II can not cross the intraocular space [143] suggesting that the systemic RAS most likely influences the intraocular RAS through the RPE.

Ang II mediates its biological effects through the activation of AT1R and AT2R receptors. It is, however, through AT1R activation that Ang II elicits most of its well known effects, including vasoconstriction, electrolyte homeostasis, fibrosis, inflammation and proliferation. In the eye, AT1R activation has been implicated in the pathogenesis of many ocular disorders such as diabetic retinopathy [144,145], neovascularization in hypoxic-induced retinopathies [146-148] and age-related macular degeneration [59,60,149]. We postulate that the interaction of Ang II with AT1R, one of the most important oxidative stress inducer: a) induces blebs formation through reactive oxygen intermediate (ROS) production by activation of NADPH promoting bleb accumulation under the RPE as BLD and b) increases MMP-2 activity, MMP-14, and basigin, major mediator of ECM turnover through MAPK phosphorylation, and pro-inflammatory monocyte chemoattractant protein-1 (MCP-1) production through NF-kB activation by RPE stimulating RPE basement membrane breakdown and infiltration of pro-inflammatory macrophages to sub-RPE deposit areas, where they will scavenge, release inflammatory mediators, growth factors or other substances, which may promote complications and progression to CNV [37,51,62]. Moreover, we propose that Ang II decreases TNFSF15, an anti-angiogenic cytokine expressed in inflammatory diseases, altering the balance between TNFSF15 and VEGF required for normal angiogenesis.

7. Oxidative injury to the RPE

As mentioned previously, a substantial body of literature suggests a role for oxidant injury to the RPE as a putative mechanism in the pathogenesis of AMD and addresses the protective actions of anti-oxidant. Although intuitively obvious, oxidant injury can induce either lethal responses, leading to cell death, or nonlethal responses inducing a functional change from baseline compatible with continued life of the cell but leading to dysfunction of the tissue or organ. Most studies focus on oxidant-mediated death of RPE [150-153]. Yet, RPE death (so-called geographic atrophy) is a very late stage of dry AMD, resulting from a very chronic and progressive process. Subretinal deposits and thickening of BrM, the hallmarks of early AMD, develop decades before the RPE cells actually die. Therefore, nonlethal cellular responses to RPE oxidant injury must contribute to early AMD.

Oxidative modifications in key cellular molecules such as DNA, carbohydrates, cellular proteins and cell membranes can often produce a cytotoxic chain reaction that contributes to the pathogenesis of many diseases [154-156]. However, we believe that oxidative damage to cell membranes and cellular proteins is more important in AMD.

RPE cell membranes are highly susceptible to lipid peroxidation. Phospholipids in RPE and photoreceptor membranes are especially rich in polyunsaturated fatty acid (PUFAs), including the ω-3 fatty acid docosahexanoic acid and the ω-6 fatty acid arachadonic acid. The presence of both types of PUFAs in phagocytosed photoreceptor outer segments renders the RPE cell membrane especially susceptible to lipid peroxidation and blebbing [157,158]. Cellular proteins are also important targets of oxidant-induced modification. Typical chemical modifications include breakdown of disulfide bonds, tyrosylation, acetylation and many other biochemical changes that can alter function of the molecule [159]. Accordingly, several well-described pathways exist to remove these damage biomolecules [160]. Although any cellular protein is potentially susceptible, the actin cytoskeleton is especially vulnerable to oxidant-induced damage.

Although oxidants derived from blue-light exposure, inflammation, or endogenous metabolism are more frequently implicated in RPE injury, we have also hypothesized that environmental toxicants and various hormones and other plasma-derived molecules related to systemic health cofactors serve as oxidants to contribute to deposit formation. We embrace the pathogenic paradigm based on the response-to-injury hypothesis which proposes that sub-RPE deposits originate from RPE-derived cell membrane blebs and dysregulation of ECM turnover induced by chronic nonlethal injury to the RPE in response to oxidative damage and propose that cigarette smoking-related hydroquinone and Ang II-induced hypertension contributes to the pathogeneis of AMD by causing oxidative damage to the RPE.

7.1. Nonlethal cell derived microparticles

Cell derived microparticles are considered to be microvesicles released through the process of exocytic budding of the plasma membrane following stimulation of different cell types [161, 162]. There are two well-known cellular processes that can lead to the formation of microparticles: chemicals and physical cell activation, and apoptosis [163,164]. Mild injuries inflected to the retina elicit a cellular response in the RPE consisting in pinching off small areas of the plasma membrane, which renders small microvesicles called blebs [165] (Fig. 5). The reason(s) behind membrane blebbing remains unknown, although it has been postulated to be an attempt to discard damaged cellular constituents by the RPE cell [14]. Nonlethal cell membrane blebbing was first introduced 30 years ago as a possible pathogenic mechanism in drusen formation [38, 166,167]. Blebbing is an early morphologic sign of cell injury which occurs immediately after exposure to a wide variety of toxic agents. However this process is different from lethal blebbing and apoptosis [168-170]. As mentioned previously, under prolonged injury, blebs may accumulate between the RPE and the basal lamina underneath this cell monolayer. Based on this concept, a plausible role for blebs in the pathogenesis of dry AMD has been suggested as a likely contributor to build-up of the sub-RPE deposits, which are characteristic of the early stages of this disorder [14].

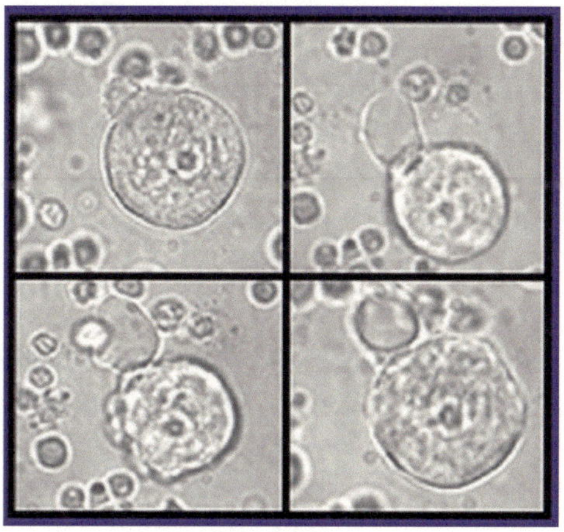

Figure 5. Plasma membrane microvesicles (blebs).

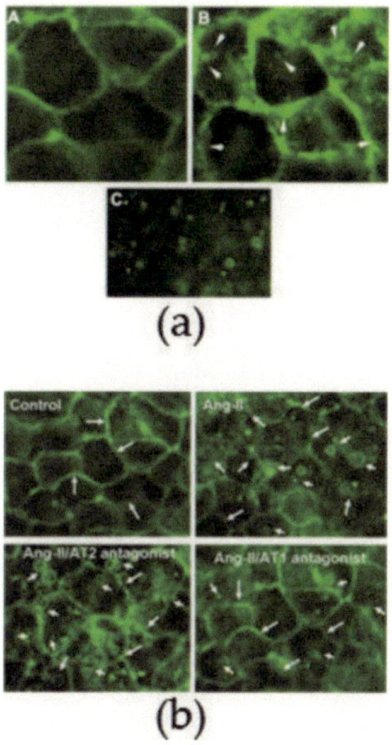

Figure 6. (a) Induction of membrane blebs in ARPE-19 cells by hydroquinone-induced cellular stress. ARPE-19 cells expressing GFP at the plasma membrane (A) were exposed to HQ (100 μM) for 6 h (B). Cells were observed immediately under epifluorescence microscope (magnification, x40). The figure shows GFP localized to the membrane and the presence of membrane blebs (white arrowheads) after HQ treatment. A detailed view of the blebs that accumulated in the conditioned medium after HQ treatment is shown (C). (b) Induction of cellular changes in ARPE-19 cells by Ang II. Fluorescent GFP-ARPE-19 derived blebs before and after exposure to Ang II (100 nM) alone or in combination with a specific Ang II receptor antagonists AT1 (CD, 100 nM) or AT2 (PD 123319, 100 nM) for 24 hours. Cells were treated and observed immediately under epifluorescent microscope. White arrows show GFP localized to the membrane. White arrowheads show the presence of membrane blebs.

Using a genetically modified human RPE cell line containing fluorescent protein anchored to the inner leaflet of the plasma membrane, we demonstrated nonlethal blebbing in response to oxidative stress. Bebbing can be induced by oxidant injury with blue light, myeloperoxidase (MPO), hydroquinone (Monroy D., et al., IOVS, 2001, 42(4), ARVO Abstract, 4060; Suner I.J., et al. IOVS 2004; ARVO E-Abstract 1810) [56,171], or Ang II (Fig. 6). Today, however, RPE bleb composition and potential functions remain largely unexplored.

Membrane bleb or microvesicle production stimulated by a variety of stress has been extensively described in many different cell types [172–178]. To gain a better understanding of the functional relevance of blebs in general and the pathogenic mechanism(s) involved in early AMD in particular, we investigated the identity of proteins carried by human RPE blebs. In our study, we showed the proteomics characterization of stress-induced blebs in RPE cells from human retina. We report identification of several proteins, some of them potentially involved in MMP activation, membrane lipid raft formation, and immunogenic processes (Fig. 7) [179]. In our study, we intended to gain some insight into the functional characterization of blebs to unravel some of the biological consequences of cell membrane blebbing in disease.

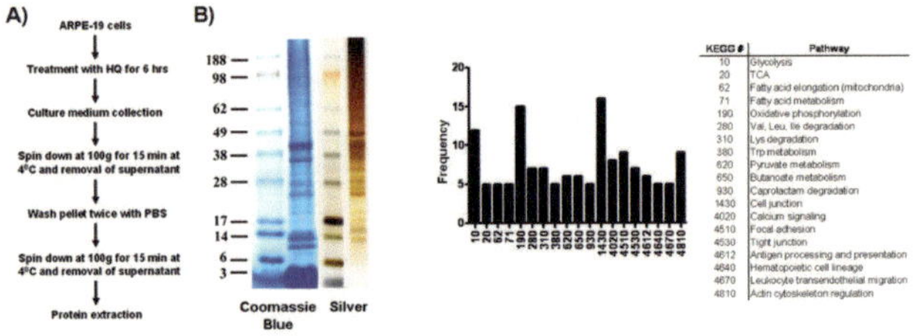

Figure 7. Isolation of blebs (left). *A,* scheme for bleb isolation. ARPE-19 cells were treated with HQ (100 μM) for 6 h. Culture medium was collected and centrifuged at 100 x g for 15 min at 4 °C. The resulting pellet was washed twice with PBS and resuspended. The resuspended pellet was centrifuged at 100 x g for 15 min at 4 °C, and the supernatant was removed. Blebs were collected and used for protein extraction. *B,* representative one-dimensional gel showing the Coomassie Blue and silver stainings of resolved proteins present in ARPE-19 blebs. Functional characterization of proteins identified in hydroquinone-induced blebs (right). The distribution profile of the proteins identified in hydroquinone-induced blebs is depicted according to functional categories. The KEGG database number and its corresponding metabolic pathway are shown. *TCA*, tricarboxylic acid cycle.

Blebbing are closely interrelated with the actin cytoskeleton [180-188]. The cytoskeleton is a dynamic structure undergoing continuous turnover by disassembly and reassembly of G-actin monomers, which are added to the active edge of a growing filament. Cytoskeletal turnover is mediated by actin polymerizing protein system (APP), which is a large system of interacting proteins. The identity of these proteins is a rapidly growing field, and includes kinases, phosphatases, cleavage proteins, and elongating proteins. Their individual specific function and regulatory interactions remain essentially unknown. However, in general, the APP functions as a coordinated system such that individual molecular regulators of cytoskeleton dynamics exert their actions on the entire APP in coordinated fashion [180-188].

Very little information is available regarding the molecules that regulate the APP system and disease pathogenesis. Interestingly, oxidant injury is an effective activator of increased cytoskeleton turnover, presumably secondary to direct oxidative changes of disulfide bonds within actin filaments [180, 189-192]. The best characterized inhibitor/ stabilizer of cytoskeleton turnover is heat shock protein 25/27 (Hsp25/27). This molecule belongs to the family of small heat shock proteins (which includes α-β crystallins) and serves a dual role as cytoskeleton stabilizer and chaperone protein [191-193].

Oxidant injury can induce a rapid upregulation of Hsp25/27 protein through the activation of presynthesized heat shock factors (hsf-1,-2,-3) which upon oxidation form trimers that become very potent transcription factors [184-189]. Upon phosphorylation, Hsp25/27 acts as an F-actin cap-binding protein, binding to the active edge of a growing microfilament, causing a transient delay in actin cytoskeleton reassembly and repair [180,181,194,195]. Transient delay in reassembly allows the unsupported plasma membrane to be forced outward by the hydrostatic forces of the cytoplasm, and a vesicle or bleb forms if cortical cytoskeleton and microfilaments do not completely reform within the outpouched membrane. Phosphorylation of Hsp25/27 is mediated through the MAP kinase cascade, but is directly phosphorylated by MAPKAP 2 kinase (MK2), which in turn is phosphorylated by p38 kinase (Figure 4) [180, 196]. Thus, oxidative stress induces profound rearrangements of the actin cytoskeleton [197, 189, 198] leading to membrane blebbing through the activation of p38 mitogen activated protein kinase (MAPK)//Heat shock protein 27 (Hsp27) pathway [190,198].

In response to stress, phosphorylated Hsp27 undergoes conformational changes and reorganizes into dimeric units [198-202]. Phosphorylated Hsp27 regulates actin filaments dynamics by repressing the ability of Hsp27 to block actin polymerization [201]. Hsp27 phosphorylation has been abundantly described in several human diseases [203]. Yet, there is a complete lack of information regarding the possible association between phosphorylated Hsp27 and AMD. Increased Hsp27 protein content along with evidence of cellular oxidative stress was reported in human eyes with AMD, but Hsp27 phosphorylation was not investigated [204]. Therefore, we believe that Hsp27 is an important mediator of RPE response to hydroquinone-induced oxidative damage, which may contribute to injury-induced actin rearrangement and blebbing. We studied the phosphorylation of Hsp27 in RPE from human eye donors and found that the RPE constitutively express phosphorylated Hsp27, and that its expression is increased in patients with dry AMD (Fig. 8) [205] providing novel evidence that phosphorylated Hsp27 may play a major role in the pathogenesis of AMD.

We reported that human RPE cells constitutively express high levels of Hsp27 which were regulated by oxidative-mediated injury and that Hsp27 is expressed in extruded blebs confirming that Hsp27 plays a role in actin filaments dynamics [205, 206]. We also addressed the question whether hydroquinone-induced oxidative injury can activate different MAPK pathways of any posttranslational modifications such as dimerization or phosphorylation of Hsp27 known to regulate F-actin polymerization. Our previous observations were extended by showing that exposure of RPE cells to cigarette smoke-derived hydroquinone non lethal injury induces the transcriptional activation of Hsp27, accumulation of Hsp27 dimers and a rapid phosphorylation of Hsp27 as well as actin rearrangements inton aggregates and membrane blebbing (Fig. 9) [205]. These results together with the observation that SB203580, a specific pharmacologic inhibitor of p38 kinase activity [207], efficiently blocked Hsp27

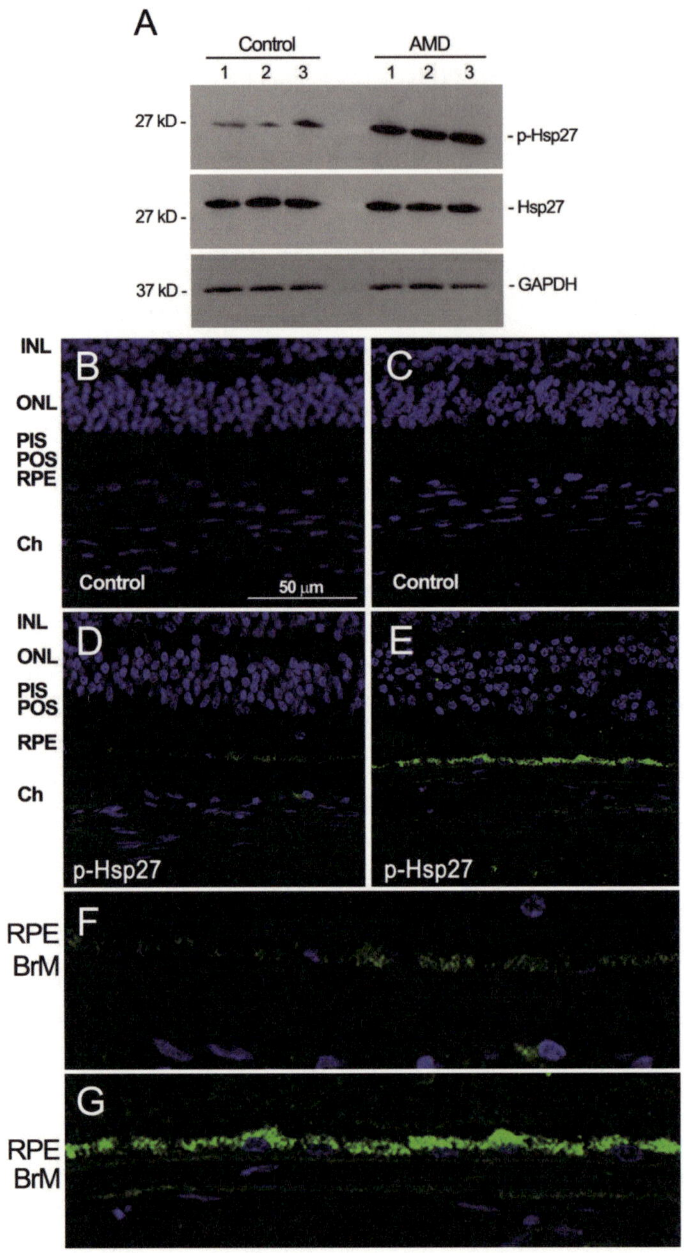

Figure 8. Increased phosphorylated Hsp27 (p-Hsp27) expression in human RPE from patient donors with dry AMD. A: Representative Western blot for p-Hsp27, total Hsp27 and GAPDH on RPE lysates from 3 donors with dry AMD and 3 controls with no known history of eye disease. B-G: Representative immunofluorescent double staining of p-Hsp27 (green) and nuclei (bleu) in retina sections from human donor eyes with no known eye disease (D), and human donor eyes with dry AMD (E). Negative controls were generated by omission of the primary antibody (B, C). Higher magnification showing RPE and BrM in control (F) and AMD (G) patients. Sections were analyzed using confocal microscopy (magnification x40 and x400). INL, inner nuclear layer; ONL, outer nuclear layer; PIS, photoreceptor inner segments; POS, photoreceptor outer segments; RPE, retinal pigment epithelium; Ch, choroid; BrM, Bruch's membrane.

phosphorylation as well as actin cytoskeleton remodeling and blebs formation in response to hydroquinone in RPE cells, strongly suggest that p38 MAPK pathways activation by hydroquinone modulates F-actin aggregates formation and membrane blebbing through Hsp27 phosphorylation. Our findings are in agreement with prior studies reporting p38 MAPK signaling pathway as an upstream mediator in oxidative stress-induced actin reorganization and Hsp27 phosphorylation [190, 198-200, 208].

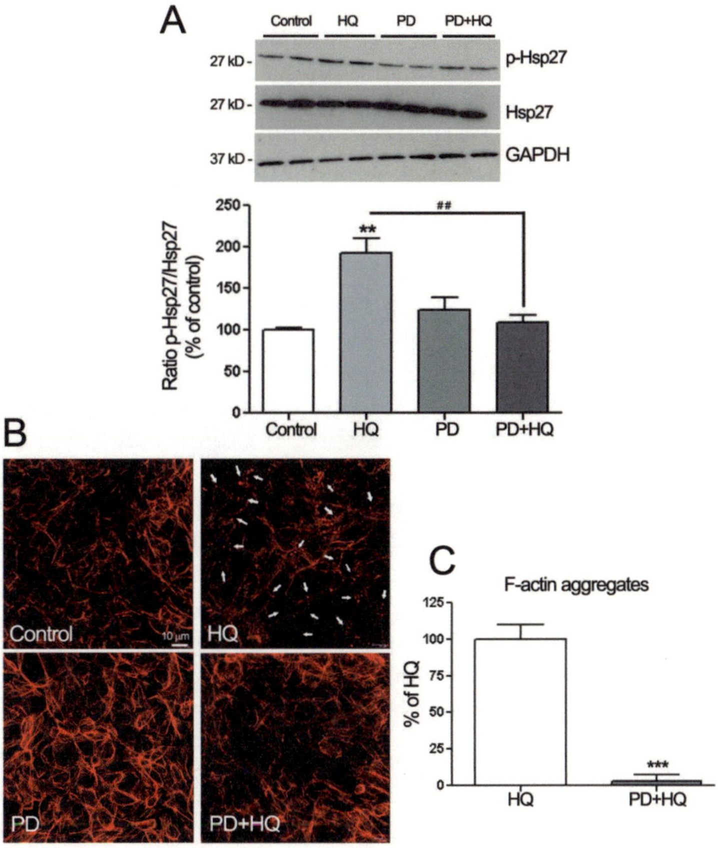

Figure 9. Inhibition of ERK MAPK pathway blocks hydroquinone (HQ)-induced Hsp27 phosphorylation and focal aggregates formation. A: Abrogation of HQ-induced Hsp27 phosphorylation by PD98059. Confluent serum-starved ARPE-19 cells were pretreated for 1 hour with 40μM of ERK inhibitor PD98059 (PD), and then exposed to 100μM HQ for 5 min. Total Hsp27, p-Hsp27 and GAPDH protein expression was evaluated by Western blot analysis. Top: Western blot from a representative experiment. Numbers on the left represent protein molecular mass in kilodaltons (kD). p-Hsp27 protein expression was normalized to total Hsp27 protein. Bottom: average densitometry results of three independent experiments run in duplicate. Data are expressed as percentage of control and are means ± SE. **$p< 0.01$ versus control; ##$p< 0.01$ versus HQ alone. B: Decreased formation of F-actin aggregates showed by staining for F-actin in ARPE-19 cells pretreated for 1 hour with or without 40μM of PD and then exposed to 100μM HQ for 6 hours. Cells were stained with rhodamine-phalloidin and examined by confocal microscopy using magnification x40. White arrowheads show formation of focal aggregates. C: Quantification of F-acting aggregates from three independent experiments run in duplicate. Data are expressed as percentage of HQ-treated cells and are means ± SE. ***$p < 0.001$ versus HQ-treated cells.

Several reports have shown that PP2A is involved in Hsp27 dephosphorylation [209, 210] and that oxidative stress causes extracellular-signal-regulated kinases (ERK) phosphorylation and reorganization of actin cytoskeleton in RPE cells [211]. Using okadaic acid as an inhibitor of Hsp27 dephosphorylation by PP1 and 2A, we observed an increase in Hsp27 phosphorylation in hydroquinone-stimulated RPE cells as well as F-actin reorganization and blebs formation [205]. Moreover, we demonstrate that Hsp27 phosphorylation and F-actin aggregates formation is almost completely abolished in cells transfected with siRNA against Hsp27 following treatment with hydroquinone [205].

As mentioned above ERK cascade participates in numerous intracellular signaling pathways in response to environmental stimuli, such as oxidative stress [211]. Our study also show that treatment with hydroquinone led to a robust activation of ERK signaling pathway in ARPE-19 cells as well as in mice. These results together with the observation that PD98059, a specific pharmacologic inhibitor of MEK, completely abolished Hsp27 phosphorylation as well as actin cytoskeleton remodeling in response to hydroquinone, strongly suggest that ERK is also a key upstream activator of hydroquinone-induced Hsp27 phosphorylation in RPE cells [205] (Fig 9). Our results not only showed that kinetics of p38 and ERK phosphorylation correlated well with that of Hsp27, but also that Hsp27 phosphorylation and F-actin aggregates formation were decreased after inhibition of either p38 or ERK signaling cascades. These observations suggest that p38 as well as ERK MAPK pathways are required for the optimal activation of Hsp27 leading to F-actin rearrangement and bleb formation in RPE cells in response to hydroquinone. Taken together,these data establish; a) a direct correlation between levels of phosphorylated Hsp27 and actin cytoskeleton reorganization in response to hydroquinone-induced oxidative injury in human RPE cells; b) present ERK as a novel upstream positive regulator of Hsp27 and actin aggregates formation in response to hydroquinone-induced oxidative injury in RPE cells; and c) give support to a key role of phosphorylated Hsp27 in the regulation of F-actin filaments dynamics and blebs formation following hydroquinone-induced oxidative stress in RPE cells. Given that there is no effective treatment for dry AMD, this study highlights Hsp27 as a potential, disease-related protein as well as biochemical pathways for potential therapeutic strategies.

In addition to Hsp27/Hsp25, other important molecules such as small GTPases protein superfamily (RAS and Ral) have been involved in the regulation of the actin polymerizing protein system and oxidative stress [212,213]. Membrane blebbing is RhoA-, Rho kinase (ROCK)-, and myosin light chain kinase (MLCK)-dependent, and blebs are devoid of actin, mDia1 and Arp2/3 [214]. Rals are small G proteins that cycle between an active GTP-bound state and an inactive GDP-bound state [215]. Ral GDP dissociation stimulator (RalGDS) was found to be an effector of Ras [216-218] and highly specific for RalA and RalB, whereby it facilitates the exchange of GDP for GTP on Rals [216,219,220]. Moreover, it has been demonstrated that RalGDS forms a cytosolic complex with β-arrestin, and that in response to formyl-Met-Leu-Phe (fMLP) receptor stimulation, RalGDS is released from β-arrestin and translocates to the plasma membrane.

RhoA is an additional small G protein that is implicated in regulating plasma membrane dynamics. RhoA is activated by Ang II and is necessary for AT1 receptor-induced stress fiber formation [221]. The proteins ROCK and mDia1 are both RhoA effectors and have been shown to play a role in changes in actin cytoskeletal reorganization. RhoA acts through ROCK to form stress fibers [240], and ROCK has been shown to be involved in cell contraction induced by Ang II [222]. mDia1 is a member of the ubiquitous formin protein family. These proteins are activated by interaction with Rho GTPases and are then able to mediate actin polymerization [223]. Overexpression of the GTP-Rho binding domain of mDia1 causes spontaneous membrane blebbing [224].

Ang II-stimulated membrane bleb formation involves RhoA. Furthermore, membrane blebbing activated by Ang II through AT1 receptor activation is attenuated in the presence of the β-arrestin amino-terminal domain, Ral GDP dissociation stimulator (RalGDS) β-arrestin binding domain, and short interfering RNA (siRNA) depletion of β-arrestin2 [225]. In addition, the inhibition of the downstream RhoA effectors ROCK and MLCK effectively attenuated AT1 receptor-mediated membrane blebbing. Thus, membrane blebbing in response to AT1 receptor signaling was dependent on β-arrestin2 and was mediated by a RhoA/ROCK/MLCK-dependent pathway providing evidence that agonist stimulation of AT1 receptor leads to plasma membrane blebbing responses by activation of RhoA and subsequent coupling to the ROCK/MLCK pathway [225].

Cytoplasmic actin aggregates were observed after nonlethal blebbing, but not with lethal oxidant injury. Interestingly, activation of the AT1 receptor with Ang II resulted in the rapid formation of ROS and membrane blebs at early time points of Ang II stimulation that cease within 60 min of Ang II stimulation (Marin-Castano., et al., IOVS, 2001, 42(4), ARVO Abstract, 4060). Further, Ang II-enhanced ROS production and blebbing was prevented by pre-treatment of RPE with the AT1 receptor blocker, which attenuates oxidative stress [226]. However, RPE derived blebs after Ang II were bigger than those seem when RPE cells were exposed to blue light, MPO, or hydroquinone. Moreover, formation of RPE-membrane blebs induced by Ang II occurred earlier than with the other oxidants we studied. Therefore, we believe that Rho-kinase pathway could be implicated as an important mediator of RPE response to Ang II-induced oxidative damage instead of Hsp27/Hsp25/p38/ERK pathway.

In conclusion, characterization of the molecular mechanism(s) by which hydroquinone and the AT1 receptor regulates the actin cytoskeleton and plasma membrane dynamics will be essential for modulating the degree of blebbing in vitro and deposit formation in vivo for potential therapeutic strategies.

Another injury response relevant to early AMD is imbalance in ECM turnover. The normal anatomy and physiology of ECM in most tissues requires continuous turnover of matrix components by a tightly regulated balance in the production of matrix molecules like collagen, laminin, matrix metalloproteinases (MMPs), and tissue inhibitors of metalloproteinases (TIMPs) [227,228]. Matrix metalloproteinases (MMPs) are a family of at least 20 zinc endopeptidases that take part in the regulation of cell matrix composition by cleaving basal lamina and ECM proteins. MMPs can be secretory or cell surface bound. Under normal conditions, MMP activity is required for tissue remodeling, but altered MMP activity has been reported in disease. Most MMPs are secreted as inactive pro-proteins but get activated when cleaved by extracellular proteinases. Interestingly, one of the targets of MMP activity is the ECM molecules in BrM.

It has been shown that relatively small dysregulation in the relative production of MMPs, TIMPs, and collagen types I and IV [227,228] may lead to net changes in the ECM, including thickening and deposit formation [228,231]. Accordingly, dysregulated turnover of ECM is a major mechanism of disease pathogenesis in many tissue sites, including renal disease, atherosclerosis, lung disease, and others [228-231]. Unfortunately, minimal information is available concerning normal turnover in healthy BrM or imbalanced turnover in AMD.

Ample evidence supports the idea that MMPs and their tissue inhibitors TIMPs play an important role in AMD. The RPE is capable of producing many ECM components such as MMP-2, MMP-14, Basigin, also known as EMMPRIN (extracellular matrix metalloproteinase inducer) or CD147, collagen, and TIMP-2 [56,171,232, 233]. MMP-2 and MMP-14 are the major RPE enzymes synthesized for the degradation of matrix type IV and I collagens, laminin, and fibronectin, which are components found in BrM [232,233]. MMP-2 is the key enzyme for ECM turnover in BrM and is synthesized as an inactive zymogen pro form (pro-MMP-2) [227]. The transmembrane metalloproteinase MMP-14 is well known to activate MMP-2 in a specific manner [233]. On the other hand, TIMP-2 may inhibit the cleavage of pro-MMP-2 into MMP-2 [228]. Based on these data our research focuses on MMP-2, MMP-14, basigin, and TIMP-2 and propose that dysregulation of MMP-2 is the primary cause for the accumulation of sub-RPE deposits that become BLD and drusen. Thus, preservation of RPE-derived MMP-2 function will prevent these events.

As mentioned before, oxidative injury to the RPE may not only produce blebbing but also dysregulated ECM turnover [5,46,47,206,234,235]. Our group has demonstrated that nonlethal oxidant injury to the RPE with hydroquinone induces a wide range of changes in gene expression, especially for those genes involved in regulation of ECM [47], and that blebs form and accumulate in the absence of activated MMP-2, which otherwise induce breakdown of types I and IV collagen present in the basement membrane of the RPE [235]. Sustained oxidant injury with hydroquinone is capable of downregulating MMP-2 activity in an in vitro system of RPE cells, correlating with an increase in bleb levels [56,171]. Also, type IV collagen accumulation, the main component of the RPE basement membrane, correlated with the absence of MMP-2 activity [56]. Accordingly, we have shown in vivo [235] that reducing MMP-2 activity leads to an increase in deposit formation by RPE cells. This allows the blebs to become trapped between the RPE cell membrane and the basement membrane to form BLD.

For the BLD deposits to progress into linear deposits ECM upregulation with MMP-2 activation is necessary for collagen and BLD deposit degradation. This will ultimately displace sub-RPE deposits into the inner layer of BrM where BLinD and drusen are histologically found. As proposed in our hypothetical model fro dry AMD, RPE-derived blebs accumulated as BLD could stimulate RPE basement membrane breakdown allowing the migration of BLD and buildup of BLiD or drusen. We postulate that various plasma-derived molecules related to systemic health cofactors (i.e., Ang II) are implicated in this stage.

As an attempt to better understand the mechanisms involved in early AMD, we investigated the proteomic profile of RPE-derived blebs induced by hydroquinone. Interestingly MMP-14 and basigin were identified in the RPE blebs [236]. Both proteins are of special relevance to the AMD pathology as they promote MMP-2 activation. Basigin, is a pleiotropic transmembrane glycoprotein [236,239]. The basigin gene (BSG) encodes for a 29 kDa protein which is prone to glycosylation increasing its molecular weight between 35 and 65 kDa [238-240]. Induction of matrix MMPs constitutes the most relevant function of basigin [240, 242-244]. A clear requirement for basigin to be glycosylated exists for MMP induction [245-247]. The fact that basigin is a prominent MMP inducer provides this protein with a putative role in normal tissue remodeling physiology and ECM pathologies other than cancer. In particular, glycosylated basigin has been reported to be necessary for maturation of the retina photoreceptor cells [248]. Within the mature eye, basigin is expressed in the RPE, Mueller cells, and in endothelial cells of blood vessels [249-252]. A known mechanism by which basigin increases the MMPs occurs at transcriptional level [253, 254]. However, shedding of basigin from the plasma membrane constitutes an additional regulatory mechanism recently proposed where basigin is transported in microvesicles which are later on degraded, releasing soluble, active basigin [255]. This proposed mechanism may permit basigin to exert its actions at distant sites. MMP-14 is an interesting candidate responsible for the basigin shedding [256-258]. Based on the cited evidence, we hypothesize a mechanistic model by which basigin and MMP-14 are carried to distal sites from the RPE where they exert their actions promoting MMP-2 activity. In addition, MMP-14 may interact with basigin releasing fully functional "soluble" basigin (Fig. 10).

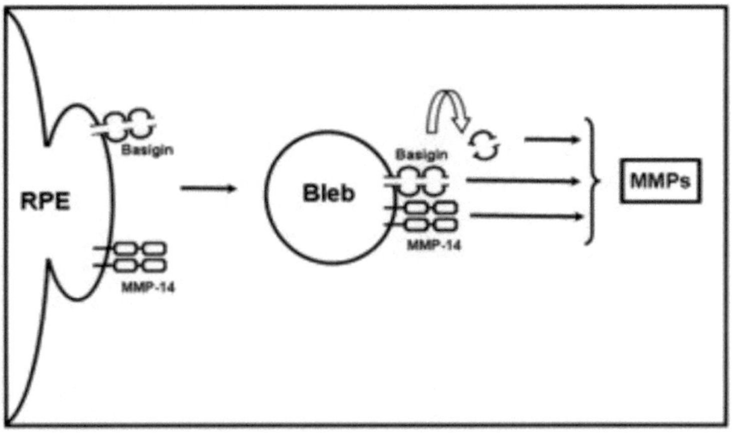

Figure 10. Mechanistic model by which basigin and MMP-14 are carried to distal sites from RPE where they exert their actions promoting MMP-2 activity.

We reported the presence of glycosylated basigin and MMP-14 in blebs, which was confirmed by Western blot and immunofluorescence staining in human control and AMD retinas (Fig. 11) [179]. Basigin and MMP-14 were confined to the RPE in normal retina, while it was widely expressed in AMD retina. In addition, our data showed that RPE cells incubated with blebs exhibit increased active MMP-2. MMP-2 activity returned to basal levels after incubation with anti-basigin and MMP-14 antibodies (Figure 10), suggesting that both proteins may play a pivotal role determining MMP-2 activity [179]. Thus, blebs accumulated under the RPE will stimulate ECM turnover increasing active MMP-2 through the action of two bleb-carried proteins, basigin and MMP-14. Therefore, we speculate that blebs may play an important role for sub-RPE to traverse RPE basement membrane. RPE are subsequently stimulated to increase synthesis of collagens and other molecules responsible for ECM turnover, affecting both RPE basement membrane and BrM. This process leads to the formation of new basement membrane under the RPE to trap these deposits within BrM. We postulate that various hormones and other plasma-derived molecules related to systemic health cofactors are implicated in this stage.

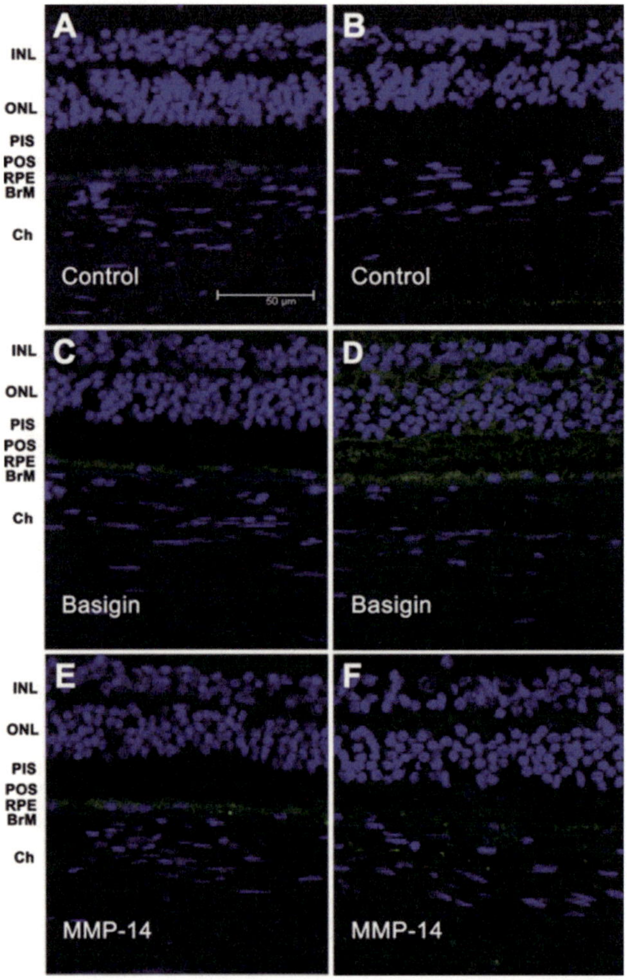

Figure 11. Immunohistochemical analysis of basigin and MMP-14 in human retina. Retina sections from human donor eyes with no known eye disease (A, C, and E) or from human donor eyes with dry AMD (B, C, and F) were stained with either mouse polyclonal anti-basigin (C and D) or mouse monoclonal anti-MMP-14 (E and F) as indicated. Negative controls were generated by omission of the primary antibody (A and B). Secondary antibodies were coupled to Alexa Fluor 488. Nuclei were stained with 4,6-diamidino-2-phenylindole dihydrochloride. Sections were analyzed under a confocal microscope. INL, inner nuclear layer; ONL, outer nuclear layer; PIS, photoreceptor inner segments; POS, photoreceptor outer segments; Ch, choroi.

8. Inflammation and angiogenesis

8.1. Inflammation: Role of cigarette smoke and angiotensin II

Another potential oxidative injury stimulus in AMD may occur during inflammation. Histopathology of AMD demonstrates that all stages of the disease, including drusen, geographic atrophy and CNV, are associated with inflammatory cells, especially macrophages [24,25,37,259,260]. One well-characterized inflammatory oxidant is myeloperoxidase (MPO), a heme protein secreted by neutrophils and macrophages that converts its substrate hydrogen peroxide into an active oxidant [206]. RPE metabolism results in high quantities of hydrogen peroxide synthesis, which by itself is a weak oxidant and is neutralized by catalase and other anti-oxidant enzyme systems [261-263]. However, in the setting of MPO release, RPE-derived hydrogen peroxide can become a powerful oxidant [171]. Macrophage-derived MPO will remain extracellular, but may initiate or potentiate the RPE injury response by catalyzing hydrogen peroxide into the formation of powerful oxidants such as hydroxyl radicals, hydroperoxides, hypochlorous acid, and tyrosyl radicals [50,264]. Among their actions, MPO-derived oxidants induce injury to the cell membrane and modify cell surface proteins and receptors [50,265,266].

Data from a number of laboratories provide compelling evidence that inflammatory and/or immune-mediated events may participate in the development of sub-RPE deposits formation and/or progression to CNV [12,24, 267-269]. Based upon available data, a new paradigm has been introduced for sub-RPE formation and its relationship to AMD. This integrated hypothesis is based largely upon the dynamic interactions between those factors that induce and sustain chronic local inflammation at the level of the RPE-BrM-choroidal interface, and those mechanisms that attenuate it. Complement and immune complexes have been identified in drusen, but their pathogenic role has not been defined. This information has been recently reviewed [24-27]. Other investigators have observed that choroidal monocytes/ macrophages are present in human specimens of both early and late AMD [24,25,27,37,259,270]. Macrophages have been detected along the choriocapillaris-side of BrM underlying areas of thick drusen or other deposits [10, 260-273] and processes from choroidal monocytes have been noted to insert into BrM deposits [260] Moreover, dentritic cells are often observed in the sub-RPE space in association with whole, or portions of, RPE cells that have been shunted into BrM, prior to the time that drusen are detectable. Therefore, macrophages and choroidal dentritic cells may be activated and recruited by locally damaged and/or sublethaly injured RPE cells. This idea is consistent with the data showing that macrophages and/or dentritic cells, and thus the innate immune system, can be activated by microenvironmental tissue damage [14,274,275]. However it remains to be determined whether drusen-associated macrophages and dentriric cells initiate a classical immune response involving T helper cells, secreted cytokines, elicit an inflammatory or complement-mediated response, or play some other role in the generation of drusen.

While it is largely recognized that macrophages accumulate in AMD lesions, there is ambiguity surrounding their role in the disease process with conflicting evidence regarding whether they might be helpful by scavenging accumulated debris and therefore protecting against CNV or harmful by stimulating CNV [100]. This might be due to the largely observational nature of human samples but also probably reflects different functions macrophages serve during distinct phases of the disease.

Inflammation is a complex process that involves local secretion of pro-inflammatory cytokines (leukocyte adhesion molecules, ICAM-1 and VCAM-1) [276,277], MCP-1 [278-282] NFκB [283-285], and growth factors (tumour necrosis factor, TNF-α, TGF-β). The key inflammatory molecule in initiating inflammatory responses may be MCP-1 [278-284] a powerful chemokine, expressed at sites of injury. Indeed, the importance of MCP-1 in inflammatory diseases is highlighted by a careful MEDLINE search for MCP-1, which readily returns more than 3000 citations following its characterization in the late 1980s. NFκB appears to control expression of MCP-1 [283-285]. After release, it activates the CCR2 chemotactic receptor to induce chemotactic responses that mediate monocyte and macrophage migration into sites of active inflammation in various diseases [286,287].

Based upon the assumption that injured RPE may serve as stimulatory factors that initiate macrophages recruitment and activation, it was determined if monocyte populations from individual AMD patients exhibited heterogeneity in terms of cytokine production in culture or in mRNA expression of freshly isolated cells, and if high levels served as a biomarker of risk for progression into neovascular AMD [51]. TNF-α expression, a potent cytotoxic and proangiogenic cytokine for wet AMD. Typically human macrophages in culture, after stimulation with RPE derived blebs produced an increase in TNF-α. However, extremely high variability in baseline TNF-α expression from isolated macrophages was observed among different subjects [51]. These results are consistent with the hypothesis that the pre-existing macrophage activation state, defined as level of cytokine or mediator expression of the circulating monocyte, might determine the negative or positive consequence of macrophage recruitment as a disease modifier. Macrophages with low expression might remove deposits safely whereas macrophages with high expression might produce mediators that contribute to disease progression.

As mentioned above, aberrant expression of chemokines occurs in a variety of diseases that have an inflammatory component. Highly specialized RPE cells play a pivotal role in the maintenance of the outer retina by secreting several cytokines including monocyte chemoattractant protein-1 (MCP-1) [288,289] which has been suggested to be implicated in the pathogenesis of AMD [290,291]. RPE cells can secrete MCP-1 in the direction of choroidal blood vessels during inflammatory responses therefore suggesting that RPE cells might promote macrophage recruitment to the choroid from circulating monocytes [292]. It was reported that MCP-1 is regulated in injured ARPE-19 cells and that free radicals might be immunostimulatory [293] providing support for the notion that injured RPE cells may induce monocyte migration.

We have investigated MCP-1 expression in RPE from patients with AMD as well as the regulation of RPE-derived MCP-1 expression following cigarette hydroquinone-mediated oxidative injury. Our data report for the first time that MCP-1 expression is markedly decreased in RPE from smoker patients with AMD [294] thereby pointing to a critical role for MCP-1 in the pathogenesis of the disease. We acknowledge that due to the nature of our study, it cannot be determined whether the altered expression of MCP-1 in human RPE lysates is a cause or consequence of the disease. However, our current findings suggest that declining

MCP-1 production by aging RPE cells may impair recruitment of macrophages/dentritic cells essential for scavenging debris which may lead to drusen formation and accumulation in AMD patients. It can be speculated that declining RPE-derived MCP-1 production resulting from cumulative exposure to oxidative damage may be an important factor that could accelerate and promote the formation of sub-RPE deposits in smokers. This theory is put forth bearing in mind the complexity of underlying cellular and molecular mechanisms involved in the inflammatory response and with the acknowledgment that numerous AMD genotypes may exist. Therefore, we fully recognize that only some aspects of the proposed hypothesis may be involved in any given AMD genotype.

Based on the above hypothesis, we have evaluated the possibility that hydroquinone-induced oxidative stress might regulate MCP-1 expression in the RPE. We showed that prolonged exposure to hydroquinone-induced oxidative injury downregulated MCP-1 production by ARPE-19 cells and RPE/choroids from C57BL/6 mice [294]. An earlier study by Joly et al is in line with our observations showing a decline in MCP-1 gene expression in retinas of mice exposed to light-induced oxidative damage for several days [294]. Our observations suggest that sustained exposure to hydroquinone might impair RPE-derived MCP-1-mediated scavenging macrophages and dentritic cells recruitment and phagocytosis which might lead to incomplete clearance of proinflammatory debris trapped between the RPE and its BrM. On the other hand, our preliminary date show that RPE-derived blebs activate RPE MCP-1 production (unpublished data), suggesting that when significant BLD will have already formed, RPE-blebs and other debris will activate MCP-1 secretion by RPE leading to infiltration of proangiogenic macrophages to sub-RPE deposit areas, where they will scavenge, relate more cytokines and mediators, and amplify the process leading to progression of drusen to CNV in smoker patients with AMD.

Angiotensin II is not only a potent vasoconstrictor which elevates arterial blood pressure, but also a powerful pro-inflammatory cytokine, chemokine and growth factor [276, 283-285,295], which mediates the activation of inflammatory mechanisms involved in age-related diseases [296,297]. There is accumulating evidence that Ang II can cause target organ damage by facilitating inflammatory and growth responses through activation of NFκB [276, 283-285], the key nuclear transcription factor in inflammatory and fibrotic diseases. Activation of NFκB by Ang II may stimulate transcription of numerous inflammatory genes, including MCP-1, RANTES (Regulated on Active Normal T cell Expressed and Secreted) and interleukin (IL)-6, TNF-α and TGF-β [276,283-285]. The view that MCP-1 is one of the most important chemokines in Ang II-induced inflammatory responses is supported by numerous studies, although the mechanisms by which Ang II increases MCP-1 expression and production are still not well understood [279,283-285]. In a rabbit model of atherosclerosis, ACE1 inhibitor quinapril inhibited NFκB activity, expression and production of MCP-1 and neointimal macrophage infiltration at the injured sites [283]. In Ang II-induced hypertensive rats, vascular MCP-1 mRNA expression increased almost four-fold, which was significantly reduced by normalization of hypertension by the non-specific vasodilator hydralazine, but the effects of AT1 receptor blockade were not studied [301]. However, in a different study, Ang II enhanced expression of MCP-1 mRNA and protein production in rat vascular smooth muscle cells in a dose- and time-dependent fashion, and these effects were mediated by AT1 receptors involving the Rho-kinase pathway [298]. In mice, Wu et al. [299] showed that the AT1 receptor antagonist valsartan, at a dose that did not influence systolic blood pressure, significantly reduced the expression of MCP-1 along with other inflammatory genes such as TNF-α, IL-6, IL-1β and monocyte/macrophage infiltration in injured vessels. Interestingly, the effects of valsartan on MCP-1 expression were attenuated in AT2 receptor-deficient mice, suggesting that both AT1 and AT2 receptors are involved.The advantage of using a lower dose of AT1 receptor blockers is that the treatment does not reduce systolic blood pressure to the normotensive level, but retains clinical efficacy in inhibiting MCP-1 expression and improving cardiac function and mortality. Accordingly, the beneficial effects of the AT1 receptor blockers may be explained by a mechanism other than high blood pressure. A direct effect of Ang II on MCP-1 expression and production may be implicated [295].

Finally, the signalling mechanisms by which Ang II increases MCP-1 expression and production and induces end-organ damage remain to be elucidated. As mentioned previously, there is mounting evidence that NFκB may be one of the most important nuclear transcription factors that mediates Ang II-stimulated MCP-1 expression and production [276,283-285]. However, the signalling pathways by which Ang II directly or indirectly activates NFκB, which is then translocated into the nucleus to mediate MCP-1 transcription and synthesis, remain largely unknown. A local RAS may be activated in most, if not all, diseases with consequently increased tissue or intracellular Ang II. Binding of extracellular Ang II to cell surface AT1 receptors may stimulate MCP-1 mRNA expression through activation of different intracellular signalling cascades, likely involving protein kinase C-activated intracellular calcium mobilization [300], tyrosine kinase and mitogen-activated protein kinase [301], phospholipase A_2 [302] and redox-sensitive NADH/NAD(P)H oxidase [301]. Future studies further addressing these important issues could improve our understanding of the potential role of pro-inflammatory cytokines and chemokines in mediating Ang II-induced target organ damage and assist in further development of novel drugs to prevent and treat these diseases.

Even if it has been suggested that increased MCP-1 expression may be a key mediator between Ang II and retinal damage in hypertensive patients, MCP-1 expression has not been investigated in RPE from hypertensive patients with AMD nor has been the regulation of RPE-derived MCP-1 expression following Ang II-mediated injury.

On the basis of our preliminary data and those of others, we have proposed a molecular inflammatory hypothesis for AMD that describes a central role for the redox-sensitive NF-κB in modulating the gene expression of MCP-1. Many studies have provided experimental evidence indicating that NF-κB can be activated by oxidative stress [303-305] and that the antioxidant may have beneficial effects on vascular inflammation that occurs in other age-related diseases [306,307]. Thus, we proposed that Ang II will active RPE MCP-1 production leading to recruitment of macrophages to sub-RPE deposit areas, where they will scavenge, release more cytokines and mediators, and amplify the process promoting complications, especially CNV formation. Our preliminary data indicate that expression of MCP-1, key mediators pertinent to inflammation is markedly increased in cultured human RPE cells in response to Ang II (Fig. 12). Moreover, our data indicate that the increase in MCP-1 mRNA and protein secretion by RPE was through AT1 receptors activation (Fig. 12), highlighting such pro-inflammatory role of Ang II and their mechanism. These observations may have strong implications for the drusen progression to CNV in hypertensive patients with dry AMD.

Future studies addressing whether or not Ang II directly or indirectly activates NFκB and the signalling pathways could improve our understanding of the potential role of Ang II in the progression of dry AMD to CNV.

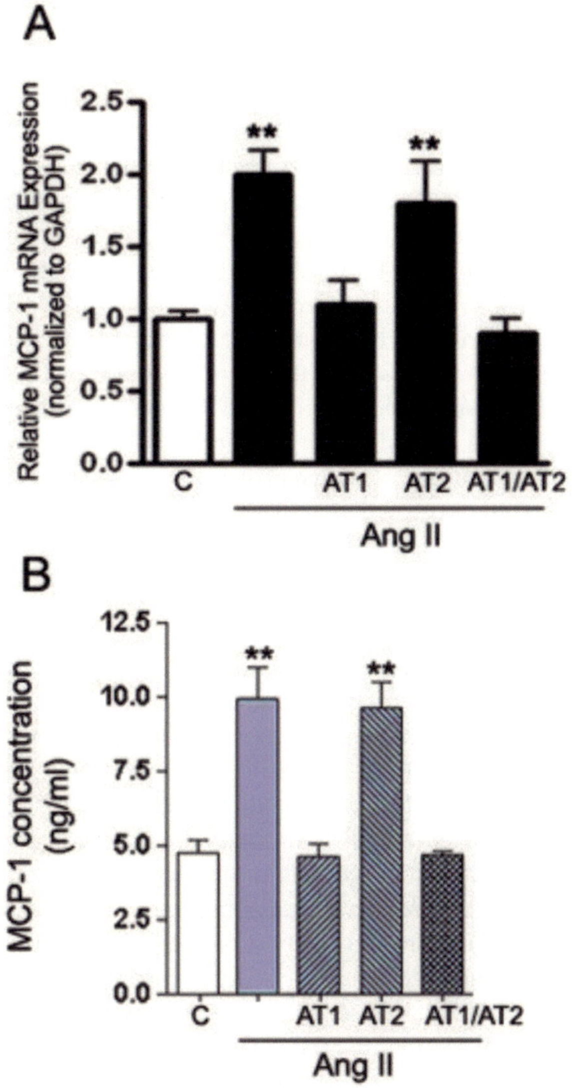

Figure 12. Ang II upregulated MCP-1 protein expression (A) and secretion (B) through Ang II receptor 1 (AT1) activation in RPE cells. Human ARPE-19 cells were incubated with Ang II alone (100 nM) for 24 hours or in combination with candesartan (CD, 100 nM), an AT1 receptor antagonist, or PD123319 (PD, 100 nM) an Ang II type 2 receptor antagonist for 30 min before Ang II stimulation, then washed with PBS and incubated in assay medium (0.1% FBS) for 24 hours. Supernatants and cell homogenates were collected to assess MCP-1 mRNA expression by real-time PCR and protein secretion by ELISA. Results are expressed as mean±SEM. **P<0.01, statistically significant difference compared with the control

Because hypertension has been unequivocally linked to the pathogenesis of AMD, it can be speculated that increase in RPE-derived MCP-1 production resulting from exposure to Ang II may be an important factor that could accelerate and promote the progression of early AMD to CNV. This theory is put forth bearing in mind the complexity of underlying cellular and molecular mechanisms involved in the inflammatory response.

8.2. Angiogenesis: Role of cigarette smoke and angiotensin II

Angiogenesis is a highly complex biological process that involves a delicate balance between numerous stimulators and inhibitors, each regulated by multiple control systems. CNV-related angiogenesis requires an alteration in the concentration of molecules that stimulate or inhibit growth of new blood vessels [308,309]. Vascular endothelial growth factor (VEGF) constitutively produced and secreted by RPE in culture [310-318], is a major angiogenic cytokine central to the development of wet AMD [312-315].VEGF regulates endothelial cells proliferation, migration and survival [315]. Interestingly, secretion of VEGF by RPE cells is polarized towards BrM [250]. There is ample clinical evidence that VEGF expression is increased in surgically excised AMD-associated choroidal neovascular membranes [315-317]. Eyes with early forms of AMD have increased expression of VEGF in the RPE and the vitreous of eyes with CNV have increased concentration of VEGF [315]. Similar observations have been made in animal models of CNV [311,320]. Furthermore, Reich et al reported that subretinal injection of VEGF siRNA significantly inhibited the growth of laser-induced CNV in a mouse model [318]. PEDF, a potent angiogenic inhibitor [321] secreted by RPE cells [322-324], counterbalances the effects of VEGF and modulates the formation of CNV [322,323]. A decrease in PEDF expression has been reported in eyes with AMD, therefore disrupting the critical balance between VEGF and PEDF that may lead to pathological angiogenesis and be permissive for the development of CNV [322]. PEDF levels decline in the vitreous of patients with CNV [324].

Interestinly, TNFSF15, a cytokine that belongs to the TNF superfamily, which originally was reported to be expressed exclusively in endothelial cells, and more recently in other several cell types in inflammatory diseases [325-328], could be implicated in the development of CNV. TNFSF15 is a potent inhibitor of endothelial cell proliferation, angiogenesis, and tumor growth [329] which has been involved in atherogenesis and neovascularization. Our preliminary data has shown constitutive TNFSF15 production and secretion by RPE in vitro and in vivo (Marin-Castano, unpublished results). Moreover, there is recent evidence showing down-regulation of TNFSF15 by VEGF in endothelial cells, therefore disrupting the critical balance between TNFSF15 and VEGF and leading to development of neovascularization [330]. Based on this recent evidence, it is conceivable that the balance between TNFSF15 and VEGF could be of great importance in CNV development. However, until now, there is no report in the literature examining VEGF, PEDF, and TNFSF15 expression in RPE from AMD patients or evaluating whether or not cigarette smoke-related hydroquinone and nicotine and Ang II have the potential to dysregulate the VEGF/PEDF and VEGF/TNFSF15 balance in RPE cells.

Given the critical role of VEGF and PEDF in AMD and that oxidative damage to the RPE and angiogenesis appear to be central in the pathogenesis of the disease; we studied the expression of these chemokines in RPE from smoker patients diagnosed with AMD and whether cigarette smoke-derived hydroquinone and nicotine might also regulate VEGF and PEDF expression in RPE cells.

We report that VEGF expression is increased and PEDF expression is decreased in RPE from smoker patients with AMD resulting in an increased VEGF-to-PEDF ratio [282]. A disruption in the critical balance of these opposing stimuli may be permissive for the development of wet AMD. Our findings are consistent with clinical observations describing dysregulated expression of VEGF and PEDF [315-317,321,322,324] in eyes with AMD. Oxidant-mediated RPE damage might promote abnormal angiogenesis [309]. In vitro, although oxidative injury declined the production of PEDF without significantly changing VEGF expression in ARPE-19 cells regardless of dose and duration of exposure to hydroquinone, we observed an increased VEGF-to-PEDF ratio which may favor angiogenesis [282]. These results suggest that cigarette smoke-related HQ-induced oxidative stress might impair the delicate balance between VEGF and PEDF that controls angiogenic homeostasis in the retina. Other previous reports showed that cigarette smoke extract induces VEGF expression in ARPE-19 cells [104] and that H_2O_2-induced oxidative stress increased the production of VEGF in human RPE cells [309]. The discrepancy between our in vitro findings and those earlier observations with regards to VEGF might reflect differences in cellular responses in the setting of different types of oxidant-mediated injury.

The endogenous angiogenic inhibitors are believed to be essential for maintaining the homeostasis of angiogenesis in the retina. Given the evidence that PEDF is an important negative regulator of angiogenesis, lower levels of PEDF is strongly suggestive of a decreased anti-angiogenic activity that may lead to the initiation of angiogenesis in response to hydroquinone-induced oxidative stress. However, we do not rule out the possibility that a decreased level of inhibitory factor PEDF by itself may not be sufficient for inducing the angiogenic switch leading to CNV. Reciprocal increase in stimulatory VEGF might also be needed. In fact, a longer more sustained exposure to hydroquinone might be necessary to induce VEGF expression in ARPE-19 cells. Furthermore, angiogenesis is a highly complex and tightly orchestrated multistep process involving extensive interplay between multiple angiogenic factors. It is therefore possible that several other molecules besides VEGF and PEDF regulated by hydroquinone might permit the development of abnormal angiogenesis. In vivo, we observed elevated expression of VEGF and PEDF protein in RPE/choroids from HQ-treated mice which translated into an enhanced VEGF-to-PEDF ratio. As stated earlier, important species-specific differences may also account for the discrepancy between human cells and mice results. In addition, one has to keep in mind that inherent in vitro and in vivo differences might explain this disparity. PEDF has multiple dose-dependent biological functions. Interestingly, it has been reported that low doses of PEDF are inhibitory but high doses can increase the development of CNV induced by laser in mice [331]. In addition, a study showed that RPE-derived VEGF upregulates PEDF expression via VEGF receptor-1 in an autocrine manner [332], therefore highlighting regulatory interactions between these two counterbalancing systems of angiogenic stimulators and inhibitors. In any case, our in vivo findings confirm that hydroquinone-induced oxidative damage is unequivocally associated with an imbalance between VEGF and PEDF in the RPE.

We also studied whether Nicotine (NT), a potent angiogenic agent abundant in second hand smoke, play a major role in the pathogenesis of wet AMD. The purpose of this study was to evaluate the expression of nicotinic acetylcholine receptors (nAchR) in the RPE and determine the effects of NT on RPE-derived VEGF and PEDF expression in the context of passive smoking. We demonstrated that cultured RPE cells constitutively expressed nAchR $\alpha3$, $\alpha10$ and $\beta1$ subunits, $\beta1$ being most prevalent (Fig. 13). nAchR $\alpha4$, $\alpha5$, $\alpha7$ and $\beta2$ subunits were detected in RPE sheets from rats, among which $\alpha4$ is the predominant subtype (Fig. 14). NT which did not, induced $\beta1$ nAchR, upregulated VEGF and downregulated PEDF expression through nAChR in ARPE-19 cells (Fig. 15). Moreover, transcriptional activation of nAchR $\alpha4$ subunit and nAChR-mediated upregulation of VEGF and PEDF were observed in RPE from rats exposed to NT [333]. Our findings confirm that NT is associated with an increased VEGF-to-PEDF ratio in RPE through nAchR in vitro and in vivo which may play a key role in the progression to wet AMD in passive smokers [333].Taken together, these data provide strong support for a key role played by hydroquinone and NT-injured RPE cells in the progression of dry AMD to CNV. We demonstrated that RPE dysfunction might lead to dysregulation of macrophage clearance function and angiogenic homeostasis as a result of oxidative damage which may trigger progression towards CNV in smoker patients with dry AMD.

As mentined previously, hypertension has been associated with the development of wet AMD in the presence of early AMD [128]. These studies make no mention of the mechanism(s) by which hypertension may induce or contribute to the progression from early AMD to CNV. Some investigators have shown that Ang II contributes to to pathological conditions such as neovascularization, atherosclerosis, and tumor [334-340]. Moreover, it has been shown that Ang II-induced angiogenesis is mediated by VEGF receptor-1 [341] and that Ang II type 2 receptor inhibits VEGF-induced migration and in vitro tube formation of human endothelial cells [342]. However, nothing is known about the regulation of TNFSF15 by Ang II in any of the tissues where it is expressed. Therefore, investigating the regulation of TNFSF15 by Ang II helped us to understand how regulation of this cytokine by Ang II could participate in the development of neovascularization in wet AMD patients with HTN. We hypothesize that hypertension through Ang II will alter the secretion of TNFSF15 release by the RPE, which may contribute to an imbalance between VEGF and TNFSF15 leading to CNV development. Our preliminary data showed that Ang II diminishes release of TNFSF15 by RPE cells through activation of both Ang II receptor subtypes and increases release of VEGF by RPE cells through activation of the AT2 Ang II receptor subtype (Marin-Castano, unpublished data), which might permit the development of abnormal angiogenesis contributing to CNV. Our study may result in the identification of TNFSF-15 as an important target to inhibit the initiation of CNV and in Ang II receptors blockade as therapeutic preventive strategy

9. Animal model for dry AMD

Animal models are extremely useful in preclinical testing of theories of disease pathogenesis and can serve to question current hypotheses and predict outcomes of therapeutic interventions. Our laboratory and others have used the C57BL/6 mouse model to evaluate mechanisms

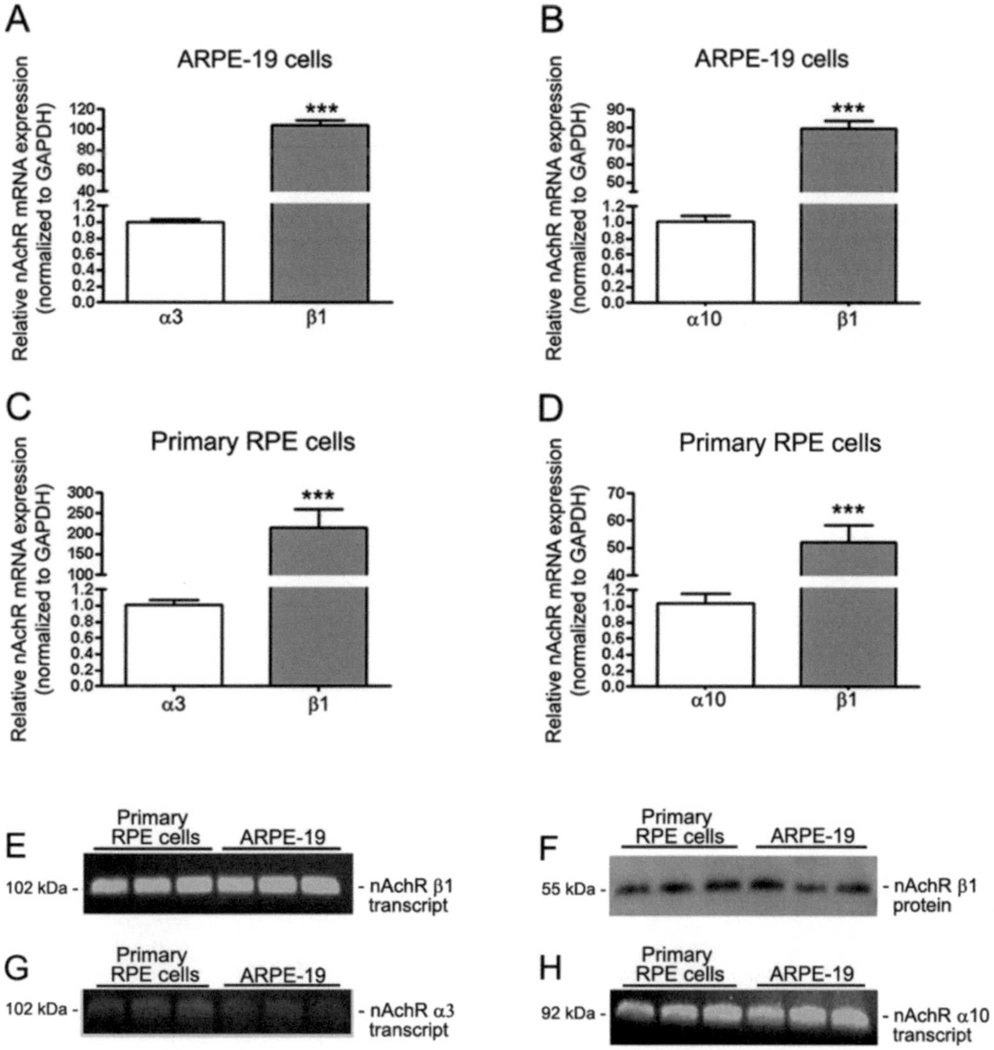

Figure 13. Human RPE cells constitutively express α3, α10 and β1 nAchR subunits. Real-time PCR demonstrated the presence of nAchR α3, α10 and β1 subunits transcripts and the prevalence of β1 subtype in confluent serum-starved (A, B, E, G, H) ARPE-19 and (C, D, E, G, H) human primary RPE cells. GAPDH was used as housekeeping gene. Real-time PCR for (E) β1, (G) α3 and (H) α10 nAchR was followed by ethidium bromide-stained agarose gel electrophoresis to visualize the products in ARPE-19 and primary RPE cells. Shown is a representative gel. Number on the left represents size of transcript in base pairs (bp). (F) Western blot analysis demonstrated the expression of the most prevalent nAchR β1 subunits in confluent serum-starved ARPE-19 and primary RPE cells. Shown is a representative gel. Number on the left represents protein molecular weight in kilodaltons (kDa).

for age, gender, diet, environmental toxins, and to text hypothesis [46,55,60,343]. Until recently, no animal models for dry AMD were available. The only available model for dry AMD and hypertension was reported by Jonas et al in 2003 [124].

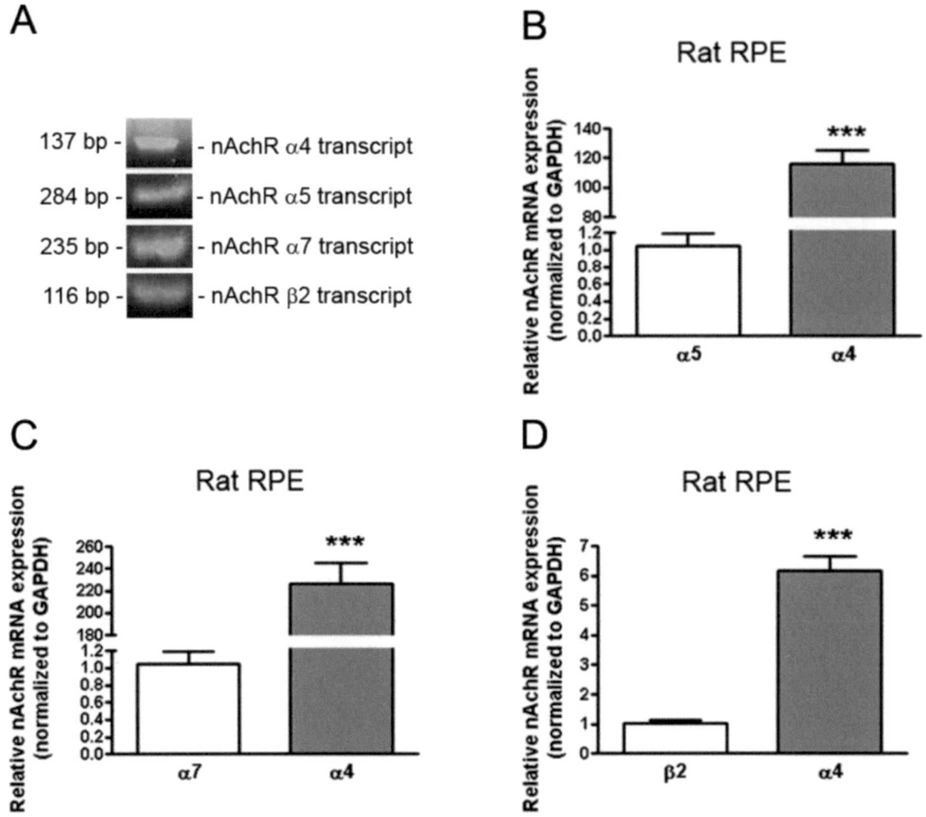

Figure 14. RPE from rats constitutively express α4, α5, α7 and β2 nAchR subunits. Real-time PCR demonstrated the presence of nAchR α4, α5, α7 and β2 subunits transcripts (A-D) and the prevalence of α4 subtype (B-D) in RPE from Sprague-Dawley rats (pooled RNA from 5 rats/lane). Real-time PCR for α4, α5, α7 and β2 nAchR isoforms was followed by ethidium bromide-stained agarose gel electrophoresis to visualize the products (A). Shown are a representative gels. Number on the left represents size of transcript in base pairs (bp). *** is $p<0.0001$.

Based on the idea that hydroquinone and arterial hypertension might influence the development and severity of drusen, we extended our in vitro data to a more physiological environment using; a) the 16-month-old or b) the 9-month-old C57BL/6 mouse model for dry AMD published by our laboratory [46,55,60,343], but providing an alternative source of oxidant stimulus by replacing exposure to blue light with exposure to hydroquinone in food [55] or drinking water [56] for 4.5 months or with Ang II alone or in combination with the AT1 receptor antagonist (candesartan) or the AT2 receptor antagonist (PD123319) for 4 weeks or 3.5 months. In addition, all mice received a regular fat diet instead of high-fat diet. We evaluated the impact of these compounds on the development of sub-RPE deposits, by using TEM.

As published previuosly, hydroquinone-treated mice had increased blood levels of hydroquinone relative to control mice that showed non detectable levels [56]. Mice not exposed to hydroquinone showed normal morphology of the RPE, BrM, and choriocapillaris endothelium (Fig. 16A). Some specimens demonstrated mild frequency of any BLD. None of the eyes in this

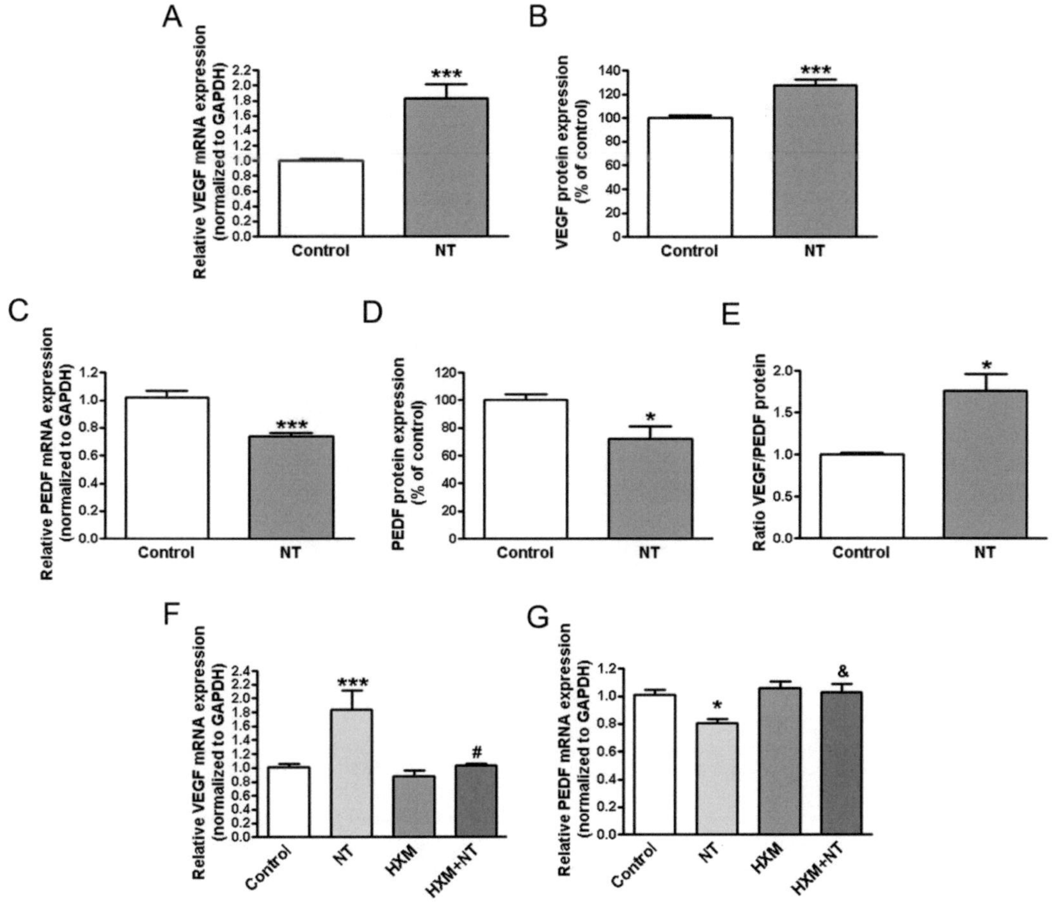

Figure 15. NT increased VEGF expression and decreased PEDF expression through nAchR in ARPE-19 cells. NT (A) increased VEGF and (C) decreased PEDF mRNA expression in ARPE-19 cells. Confluent serum-starved ARPE-19 cells were treated with NT 10^{-8}M for 72 hours. Total RNA was extracted to assess VEGF and PEDF mRNA expression by real-time PCR. GAPDH was used as housekeeping gene. NT (B) increased VEGF and (D) decreased PEDF protein expression. Concentration of VEGF and PEDF secreted in supernatants of confluent serum-starved ARPE-19 cells treated with NT 10^{-8}M for 72 hours was assessed by ELISA. (E) NT increased VEGF/PEDF protein ratio. NT-induced (F) upregulation of VEGF and (G) downregulation of PEDF mRNA expression was abolished by hexamethonium (HXM). Confluent serum-starved ARPE-19 cells were pre-incubated with HXM 10^{-5}M for 1 hour then exposed to NT 10^{-8}M for 72 hours. Total RNA was extracted to assess VEGF and PEDF mRNA expression by real-time PCR. GAPDH was used as housekeeping gene. Data are expressed as means ± SE and represent the average results of 3 to 4 independent experiments run in duplicate.* is $p<0.05$ and *** is $p<0.0001$ versus control; # is $p<0.01$ and & is $p<0.05$ versus NT alone.

group demonstrated moderate BLD. Animals exposed to hydroquinone showed pathologic changes in the RPE and BrM characterized by moderate BLD [56]. Approximately a 83% of eyes exhibited moderate BLD. The BrM was thickened, with coated vesicles, membranous profiles, and banded structures, Figs. 16B, 16C), typical of those described in some human AMD specimens [46]. Findings were of a magnitude similar to those previously observed in mice exposed to high-fat diet plus blue green light [62]. Interestingly, animals showed blebs

(Fig. 16C). In preliminary experiments, we have also demonstrated that mice receiving subconjunctival injections of hydroquinone exhibeted a rudimentary form of BLD, often demonstrating small vesicular vesicles bleblike structures (Reinoso, et al. IOVS 2005;46:ARVO E-Abstract 3010). In addition, RPE from mice exposed to hydroquinone in drinking water showed increased levels of phosphorylated Hsp25, p38 and ERK [205], suggesting that phosphorylated Hsp25 might be a key mediator in early cellular events associated with actin reorganization and bleb formation involved in sub-RPE deposits formation.

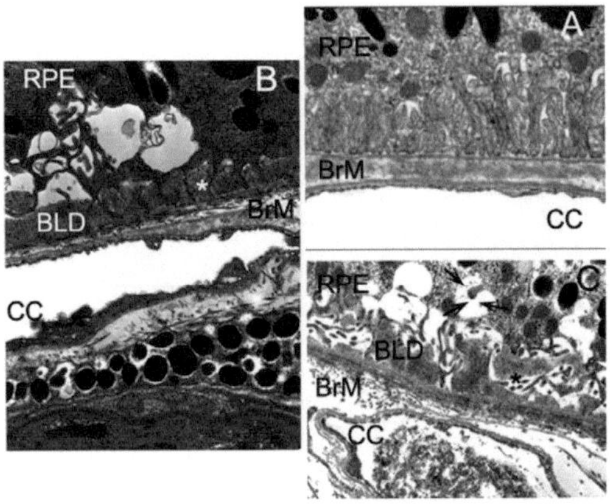

Figure 16. Transmission electron microscopy of the outer retina and choroid from a 16-month-old female mouse fed with a regular fat diet for 4 months. (A) Outer retina and choroid of a mouse fed a regular diet without oxidant showed a normal RPE, BrM, and choriocapillaris. (B) Outer retina and choroid of a mouse fed a regular diet and exposed to HQ (0.8% for 4 months) in drinking water revealed sub-RPE deposits characterized by accumulation of moderately severe BLD with dense granular material between the RPE and its basement membrane (*), compatible with a high mean severity score. The specimen, also, shows the abnormal choriocapillaris endothelium with increased thickening and loss of fenestration. (C) TEM of the outer retina and choroids from another 16-month-old female mouse fed a regular diet and exposed to HQ. The specimen shows moderately thick BLD with bandes structures (*) and occasional blebs (black arrows). CC, choriocapillaris, Magnification: (A, C) x25,000; (B) x7,200.

We used Ang II to determine whether hypertension-associated Ang II was important for ECM regulation in RPE and the development of sub-RPE deposits. We reported that Ang II-treated mice had increased blood pressure as well as plasma and ocular levels of Ang II relative to control mice [60]. Ang II also regulated AT1a and AT1b receptor mRNA expression, and the intracellular concentration of calcium $[Ca^{2+}]_I$, showing that Ang II AT1 receptor is functional. In addition, MMP-2 activity, and type IV collagen accumulation were regulated by Ang II. Concurrent administration of Ang II with the AT1 receptor blocker prevented the increase in blood pressure and rise in ocular Ang II levels, as well as the calcium and MMP-2 responses. In contrast, the type IV collagen response to Ang II was prevented by blockade of AT2 receptors, but not AT1 receptors. Plasma Ang II levels were not modified by the AT1 or AT2 receptor blockade. In addition, Ang II stimulates MMP-14, basigin, and phosphorylation of ERK, p38, and JNK in RPE sheets from mice. These effects were mediated by Ang II type 1 receptors [344].

Animals exposed to Ang II for 3.5 months revealed moderate BLD deposits. Sub-RPE changes were characterized by accumulation of moderately dense homogeneous material between the RPE and its basement membrane (Marin-Castano, unpublished data). Given that the Ang II receptors in rodents are similar to human Ang II receptors, our study help to elucidate the mechanism(s) by which Ang II receptor blockers may prevent these ECM changes important for early AMD development and provide a potential future clinical tool for the prevention of AMD. Moreover, our observations indicate that Ang II may induce the development of BLD. Thus, the results suggest the role for Ang II in ECM turnover and sub-RPE formation and propose Ang II-induced hypertension as an injury stimulus to the RPE, which may serve to explain the mechanisms that underlie pathologic BLD deposits in early AMD.

Taken together, these observations indicate that different oxidant stimuli (i.e., blue light, hydroquinone, and Ang II) may induce a common response in the RPE and that a high-fat diet is not an absolute requirement for the development of BLD. Thus, the results suggest the role for blebs in sub-RPE formation and propose hydroquinone and Ang II another oxidative injury stimulus to the RPE, which may serve to explain the mechanisms that underlie pathologic BLD deposits in early AMD.

10. Conclusions

In summary, we postulate that cigarette smoke-related and Ang II play a role in the development of dry AMD and its progression to wet AMD. Although our hypothesis remains to be proven, we have proposed new ideas and suggested different mechanisms highlighting Hsp27, MMP-2, basigin, MMP-14, MCP-1, MAPK, and TNFSF15 as potential disease-related proteins as well as biochemical pathways for potential therapeutic strategies, which might result in prevention of more severe and irreversible late stages of this dreadful disease. Our goal is to intervene promptly in the early stages of the disease so that progression to the more severe late forms of AMD can be prevented. In this respect, RPE-derived MMPs and blebs formation are potential target due to their pivotal role in stimulating drusen formation and progression into CNV. Levels of phosphorylated Hsp27, glycosilated basigin and MMP-14, as well as, MCP-1 and TNFSF15 could be markers, which may contribute and aid to the ophthalmologic community in the management of the drusen. Moreover, AT1 receptor antagonists and p38/ERK1/2 MAPK blockers could be used successfully on the prevention of sub-RPE deposits formation in selected high-risk AMD patients.

Author details

Maria E. Marin-Castaño

Department of Ophthalmology, Bascom Palmer Eye institute, University of Miami, Miami, FL, USA

References

[1] Fine, SL, & Berger, . . Age-related macular degeneration. The New England journal of medicine. 2000; 342 (7);483-492.

[2] Klein, R, Chou, C. F, Klein, B. E, Zhang, X, Meuer, S. M, & Saaddine, J. B. Prevalence of age-related macular degeneration in the US population. Archives of Ophthalmology. (2011). , 129(1), 75-80.

[3] Klein, R, Peto, T, Bird, A, & Vannewkirk, M. R. The epidemiology of age-related macular degeneration. American Journal of Ophthalmology. (2004). , 137(3), 486-495.

[4] Rein, D. B, Wittenborn, J. S, Zhang, X, Honeycutt, A. A, Lesesne, S. B, & Saaddine, J. Forecasting age-related macular degeneration through the year 2050: the potential impact of new treatments.Archives of Ophthalmology. (2009). , 127(4), 533-540.

[5] Abdelsalam, A. Del Priore L, Zarbin MA. Drusen in age-related macular degeneration: pathogenesis, natural course, and laser photocoagulation-induced regression. Survey of Ophthalmology. (1999). , 44(1), 1-29.

[6] Zarbin, M. A. Current concepts in the pathogenesis of age-related macular degeneration. Archives of Ophthalmology. (2004). , 122(4), 598-614.

[7] Abecasis, G. R, Yashar, B. M, Zhao, Y, Ghiasvand, N. M, Zareparsi, S, & Branham, K. E. Age-related macular degeneration: a high-resolution genome scan for susceptibility loci in a population enriched for late-stage disease. Am J Hum Genet. (2004). , 74, 482-494.

[8] Tuo, J, Bojanowski, C. M, & Chan, C. C. Genetic factors of age-related macular degeneration. Prog Retin Eye Res. (2004). , 23, 229-249.

[9] Rodrigues, E. B. Inflammation in dry age-related macular degeneration. Ophthalmologica. (2007). , 143-152.

[10] Oh, H, Takagi, H, & Takagi, C. The potential angiogenic role of macrophages in the formation of choroidal neovascular membranes. Invest Ophthalmol Vis Sci. (1999). , 40, 1891-1898.

[11] Liang, F. Q, & Godley, B. F. Oxidative stress-induced mitochondrial DNA damage in human retinal pigment epithelial cells: a possible mechanism for RPE aging and age-related macular degeneration. Exp Eye Res. (2003). , 76, 397-403.

[12] Donoso, L. A, Kim, D, Frost, A, Callahan, A, & Hageman, G. The role of inflammation in the pathogenesis of age-related macular degeneration. Surv Ophthalmol. (2006). , 51, 137-152.

[13] Berger, J. W, Fine, S. L, & Maguire, M. G. Age-related macular degeneration. St. Louis: Mosby, (1999).

[14] Grenn, W. R. Histopathology of age-related macular degeneration. (1999). Molecular vision, 5, 27.

[15] Bird, A. C, Bressler, N. M, Bressler, S. B, Chisholm, I. H, Coscas, G, Davis, M. D, De Jong, P. T, Klaver, C. C, Klein, B. E, Klein, R, et al. An international classification and grading system for age-related maculopathy and age-related macular degeneration. The International ARM Epidemiological Study Group. Surv Ophthalmol. (1995). Review., 39(5), 367-74.

[16] Gass, J. D. Drusen and disciform macular detachment and degeneration. Trans Am Ophthalmol Soc. (1972). , 70, 409-36.

[17] Guymer, R, Luthert, P, & Bird, A. Changes in Bruch's membrane and related structures with age. Progress in retinal and eye research. (1999). , 18(1), 59-90.

[18] Hiscott, P, Sheridan, C, Magee, R. M, & Grierson, I. Matrix and the retinal pigment epithelium in proliferative retinal disease. Progress in retinal and eye research. (1999). , 18(2), 167-190.

[19] Young, R. W. Pathophysiology of age-related macular degeneration. Survey of Ophthalmology. (1987). , 31(5), 291-306.

[20] Strauss, O. The retinal pigment epithelium in visual function. Physiol Rev. (2005). , 85, 845-881.

[21] Sheridan, C, Williams, R, & Grierson, i. Basement membranes and artificial substrates in cell transplantation. Graefe's archive for clinical and experimental ophthalmology = Albrecht von Graefes Archiv fur klinische und experimentelle Ophthalmologie. (2004). , 242(1), 68-75.

[22] Hewitt, A. T, Nakazawa, K, & Newsome, D. A. Analysis of newly synthesized Bruch's membrane proteoglycans. Investigative Ophthalmology & Visual Science. (1989). , 30(3), 478-486.

[23] Inatani, M, & Tanihara, H. Proteoglycans in retina. Progress in retinal and eye research. (2002). , 21(5), 429-447.

[24] Hageman, G. S, & Luthert, P. J. Victor Chong NH, Johnson LV, Anderson DH, Mullins RF. An integrated hypothesis that considers drusen as biomarkers of immune-mediated processes at the RPE-Bruch's membrane interface in aging and age-related macular degeneration. Prog Retin Eye Res. (2001). , 20(6), 705-732.

[25] Penfold, P. L, Madigan, M. C, Gillies, M. C, & Provis, J. M. Immunological and aetiological aspects of macular degeneration. Prog Retin Eye Res. (2001). , 20(3), 385-414.

[26] Hageman, G. S, & Mullins, R. F. Molecular composition of drusen as related to substructural phenotype. Mol Vis. (1999). Review.

[27] Anderson, D. H, Mullins, R. F, Hageman, G. S, & Johnson, L. V. A role for local inflammation in the formation of drusen in the aging eye. Am J Ophthalmol. (2002). , 134(3), 411-431.

[28] Zarbin, M. A. Age-related macular degeneration: review of pathogenesis European Journal of Ophthalmology. (1998). , 8(4), 199-206.

[29] Sarks, S, Cherepanoff, S, Killingsworth, M, & Sarks, J. Relationship of Basal laminar deposit and membranous debris to the clinical presentation of early age-related macular degeneration. Investigative Ophthalmology & Visual Science. (2007). , 48(3), 968-977.

[30] Van Der Schaft, T. L, Mooy, C. M, De Bruijn, W. C, Oron, F. G, Mulder, P. G, & De Jong, P. T. Histologic features of the early stages of age-related macular degeneration. A statistical analysis Ophthalmology. (1992). , 99(2), 278-286.

[31] Kliffen, M, Van Der Schaft, T. L, Mooy, C. M, & De Jong, P. T. Morphologic changes in age-related maculopathy. Microscopy Research and Technique.(1997). , 36(2), 106-122.

[32] Wang, L, Clark, M. E, Crossman, D. K, Kojima, K, Messinger, J. D, Mobley, J. A, & Curcio, C. A. Abundant lipid and protein components of drusen. PLoS ONE.(2010). , e10329.

[33] 33-Cherepanoff S, McMenamin P, Gillies MC, Kettle E, Sarks SH. Bruch's membrane and choroidal macrophages in early and advanced age-related macular degeneration. British Journal of Ophthalmology. 2010;94(7):918-925.

[34] la Cour MKiilgaard JF, Nissen MH. Age-related macular degeneration: epidemiology and optimal treatment. Drugs and Aging.(2002). , 19(2), 101-133.

[35] Wang, J. J, Foran, S, Smith, W, & Mitchell, P. Risk of age-related macular degeneration in eyes with macular drusen or hyperpigmentation: the Blue Mountains Eye Study cohort Archives of Ophthalmology. (2003). , 121(5), 658-663.

[36] Green, W. R, & Enger, C. Age-related macular degeneration histopathologic studies. The 1992 Lorenz E. Zimmerman Lecture. Ophthalmology. (1993). , 100(10), 1519-1535.

[37] Grossniklaus, H. E, Ling, J. X, Wallace, T. M, Dithmar, S, Lawson, D. H, Cohen, C, Elner, V. M, & Elner, S. G. Sternberg Jr P. Macrophage and retinal pigment epithelium expression of angiogenic cytokines in choroidal neovascularization. Molecular vision. (2002). , 119-126.

[38] IshibashiT; Patterson, R; Ohnishi, Y; Inomata, H; Ryan, S. Formation of drusen in the human eye. Am. J. Ophthalmol, (1986). , 101, 342-353.

[39] Donders, F. Beitrage zur pathologischen Anatomie des Auges. Graefe's Arch. Clin. Exp. Ophthalmol, (1854). , 1, 106-118.

[40] Muller, H. Anatomische beitrage zur ophthalmologie. Albrecht von Graefe Arch Ophthalmol, (1856). , 2, 1-69.

[41] Young, R. W. Pathophysiology of age-related macular degeneration. Surv Ophthalmol. (1987). , 31(5), 291-306.

[42] Farkas, T, Sylvester, V, & Archer, D. The ultrastructure of drusen. Am J Ophthalmol. (1971). , 71, 1196-1205.

[43] Feeney-burns, L, Gao, C, & Tidwell, M. Lysosomal enzyme cytochemistry of human RPE, Bruch's membrane and drusen. Invest. Ophthalmol Visual Sci. (1987). , 28, 1138-1147.

[44] El Baba, F, Green, W, Fleischmann, J, Finkelstein, D, & De La Cruz, Z. Clinicopathologic correlation of lipidization and detachment of the retinal pigment epithelium. Am J Ophthalmol. (1986). , 101, 576-583.

[45] Charras, G. T. A short history of blebbing. J Microsc. (2008). , 231, 466-478.

[46] Cousins, S. W, Espinosa-heidmann, D. G, Alexandridou, A, Sall, J, Dubovy, S, & Csaky, K. The role of aging, high fat diet and blue light exposure in an experimental mouse model for basal laminar deposit formation. Exp Eye Res, (2002). , 75(5), 543-553.

[47] Strunnikova, N, Zhang, C, Teichberg, D, Cousins, S. W, Baffi, J, Becker, K. G, & Csaky, K. G. Survival of retinal pigment epithelium after exposure to prolonged oxidative injury: a detailed gene expression and cellular analysis. Invest Ophthalmol Vis Sci. (2004). , 45(10), 3767-3777.

[48] Beatty, S, Koh, H, Phil, M, Henson, D, & Boulton, M. The role of oxidative stress in the pathogenesis of age-related macular degeneration. Surv Ophthalmol. (2000). , 45(2), 115-134.

[49] Winkler, B. S, Boulton, M. E, Gottsch, J. D, & Sternberg, P. Oxidative damage and age-related macular degeneration. Mol Vis. (1999).

[50] Chisolm GM IIIHazen SL, Fox PL, Cathcart MK. The oxidation of lipoproteins by monocytes-macrophages. Biochemical and biological mechanisms. J Biol Chem. (1999). , 274(37), 25959-25962.

[51] Cousins, S. W, Espinosa-heidmann, D. G, & Csaky, K. G. Monocyte activation in patients with age-related macular degeneration: a biomarker of risk for choroidal neovascularization? Arch Ophthalmol. (2004). , 122(7), 1013-1018.

[52] Espinosa-heidmann, D. G, Suner, I. J, Hernandez, E. P, Monroy, D, Csaky, K. G, & Cousins, S. W. Macrophage depletion diminishes lesion size and severity in experimental choroidal neovascularization. Invest Ophthalmol Vis Sci. (2003). , 44(8), 3586-3592.

[53] Marin-castano, M. E. Angiotensin II receptor expression and function in retinal pigment epithelium. Investigative Ophthalmology & Visual Science. (2004). ARVO E-Abstract)., 1811.

[54] Striker, G. E, Praddaude, F, Alcazar, O, Cousins, S. W, & Marin-castaño, M. E. Regulation of angiotensin II receptors and extracellular matrix turnover in human retinal pigment epithelium: role of angiotensin II. Am J Physiol Cell Physiol. (2008). C , 1633-46.

[55] Espinosa-heidmann, D. G, Suner, I. J, Catanuto, P, Hernandez, E. P, Marin-castano, M. E, & Cousins, S. W. Cigarette smoke-related oxidants and the development of sub-RPE deposits in an experimental animal model of dry AMD. Investigative Ophthalmology & Visual Science. (2006). , 47(2), 729-737.

[56] Marin-castano, M. E, Striker, G. E, Alcazar, O, Catanuto, P, Espinosa-heidmann, D. G, & Cousins, S. W. Repetitive nonlethal oxidant injury to retinal pigment epithelium decreased extracellular matrix turnover in vitro and induced sub-RPE deposits in vivo. Investigative Ophthalmology & Visual Science. (2006). , 47(9), 4098-4112.

[57] Elliot, S, Catanuto, P, Fernandez, P, Espinosa-heidmann, D, Korach, K. K, & Cousins, S. W. Subtype specific estrogen receptor action protects against changes in MMP-2 activation in mouse retinal pigmented epithelial cells. Experimental Eye Research. (2008). , 86(4), 653-660.

[58] Elliot, S, Catanuto, P, Espinosa-heidmann, D. G, Fernandez, P, Hernandez, E, Saloupis, P, Korach, K, & Cousins, S. W. Estrogen receptor beta protects against in vivo injury in RPE cells Experimental Eye Research.(2010). , 90(1), 10-16.

[59] Striker, G. E, Praddaude, F, Alcazar, O, Cousins, S. W, & Marin-castano, M. E. Regulation of angiotensin II receptors and extracellular matrix turnover in human retinal pigment epithelium: role of angiotensin II. American Journal of Physiology. Cell Physiology. (2008). C , 1633-1646.

[60] Praddaude, F, Cousins, S. W, Pecher, C, & Marin-castano, M. E. Angiotensin II-induced hypertension regulates AT1 receptor subtypes and extracellular matrix turnover in mouse retinal pigment epithelium. Experimental Eye Research (2009). , 89(1), 109-118.

[61] Cousins, S. W, & Csaky, K. Immunology of Age-Related Macular Degeneration J.I. Lim (Ed.), Age-Related Macular Degeneration, Marcel Dekker, Inc., New York. (2002). , 27-65.

[62] Espinosa-heidmann, D. G, Suner, I. J, Hernandez, E. P, Monroy, D, Csaky, K. G, & Cousins, S. W. Macrophage depletion diminishes lesion size and severity in experimental choroidal neovascularization. Investigative Ophthalmology & Visual Science. (2003).

[63] Esfandiary, H, Chakravarthy, U, Patterson, C, Young, I, & Hughes, A. E. Association study of detoxification genes in age related macular degeneration. Br. J. Ophthalmol. (2005). , 89, 470-474.

[64] Clemons, T. E, Milton, R. C, Klein, R, Seddon, J. M, & Ferris, F. L. Age-Related Eye Disease Study Research Group. Risk factors for the incidence of Advanced Age-Related Macular Degeneration in the Age-Related Eye Disease Study (AREDS). Ophthalmology. (2005). , 112, 533-539.

[65] Seddon, J. M, Willett, W. C, Speizer, F. E, & Hankinson, S. E. A prospective study of cigarette smoking and age-related macular degeneration in women. JAMA. (1996). , 276, 1141-1146.

[66] Tomany, SC, Wang, JJ, Van Leeuwen, R, Klein, R, Mitchell, P, Vingerling, JR, Klein, BE, & Smith, . . Risk factors for incident age-related macular degeneration: pooled findings from 3 continents. Ophthalmology. 2004;111:1280-1287.

[67] Rahman, I. MacNee W. Role of oxidants/antioxidants in smoking-induced lung diseases. Free Radical Biology and Medicine. (1996). , 21(5), 669-681.

[68] Rahman, I. MacNee W. Role of oxidants/antioxidants in smoking-induced lung diseases. Free Radical Biology and Medicine. (1996). , 21(5), 669-681.

[69] Feng, Z, Liu, Z, Li, X, Jia, H, & Sun, L. Tian C; Jia L, Liu J. Alpha-Tocopherol is an effective Phase II enzyme inducer: protective effects on acrolein-induced oxidative stress and mitochondrial dysfunction in human retinal pigment epithelial cells. J Nutr Biochem. (2010). , 21(12), 1222-1231.

[70] Jia, L, Liu, Z, Sun, L, Miller, S. S, Ames, B. N, Cotman, C. W, & Liu, J. Acrolein, a toxicant in cigarette smoke, causes oxidative damage and mitochondrial dysfunction in RPE cells: protection by (R)-alpha-lipoic acid. Invest Ophthalmol Vis Sci. (2007). , 48(1), 339-48.

[71] Takeuchi, A, Takeuchi, M, Oikawa, K, Sonoda, K. H, Usui, Y, Okunuki, Y, Takeda, A, Oshima, Y, Yoshida, K, Usui, M, Goto, H, & Kuroda, M. Effects of dioxin on vascular endothelial growth factor (VEGF) production in the retina associated with choroidal neovascularization. Invest Ophthalmol Vis Sci. (2009). , 50(7), 3410-34166.

[72] Sharma, A, Neekhra, A, Gramajo, A. L, Patil, J, Chwa, M, Kuppermann, B. D, & Kenney, M. C. Effects of Benzo(e)Pyrene, a toxic component of cigarette smoke, on human retinal pigment epithelial cells in vitro. Invest Ophthalmol Vis Sci. (2008). , 49(11), 5111-5117.

[73] Wills, N. K, & Kalariya, N. Sadagopa Ramanujam VM, Lewis JR, Haji Abdollahi S, Husain A, van Kuijk FJ. Human retinal cadmium accumulation as a factor in the etiology of age-related macular degeneration. Exp Eye Re. (2009). , 89, 79-87.

[74] Kalariya, N. M, Wills, N. K, Ramana, K. V, Srivastava, S. K, & Van Kuijk, F. J. Cadmium-induced apoptotic death of human retinal pigment epithelial cells is mediated by MAPK pathway. Exp Eye Res. (2009). , 89(4), 494-502.

[75] Wills, N. K. Sadagopa Ramanujam VM, Chang-Strepka J, Kalariya N, Lewis JR, van Kuijk, FJ. Cadmium accumulation in the aging human retina. Exp. Eye Res. (2008). , 86(1), 41-51.

[76] Pryor, W. A. Cigarette smoke radicals and the role of free radicals in chemical carcinogenicity. Environ Health Perspect. (1997). , 105(4), 875-882.

[77] Halliwell, B. Free radicals and vascular disease: how much do we know? BMJ. (1993). , 307(6909), 885-886.

[78] Winston, G. W, Church, D. F, Cueto, R, & Pryor, W. A. Oxygen consumption and oxyradical production from microsomal reduction of aqueous extracts of cigarette tar. Arch Biochem Biophys. (1993). , 304(2), 371-378.

[79] Niki, E, Minamisawa, S, Oikawa, M, & Komuro, E. Membrane damage from lipid oxidation induced by free radicals and cigarette smoke. Ann N Y Acad Sci. (1993). , 686, 29-37.

[80] Klein, R, Knudtson, M. D, Cruickshanks, K. J, & Klein, B. E. Further observations on the association between smoking and the long-term incidence and progression of age-related macular degeneration: The Beaver Dam Eye Study. Archives of Ophthalmology. (2008). , 126(1), 115-121.

[81] Solberg, Y, Rosner, M, & Belkin, M. The association between cigarette smoking and ocular diseases. Surv Ophthalmol. (1998). , 42, 535-547.

[82] Chow, C. K, Thacker, R. R, Chow, C. K, Thacker, R. R, Changchit, C, Bridges, R. B, Rehm, S. R, Humble, J, & Turbek, J. Lower levels of vitamin C and carotenes in plasma of cigarette smokers. J Am Coll Nutr. (1986). , 5(3), 305-312.

[83] Church, D. F, & Pryor, W. A. Free-radical chemistry of cigarette smoke and its toxicological implications. Environ Health Perspect. (1985). , 64, 111-126.

[84] Rahman, I. MacNee W. Role of oxidants/antioxidants in smoking-induced lung diseases. Free Radical Biology and Medicine. (1996). , 21(5), 669-681.

[85] AREDSA randomized, placebo-controlled, clinical trial of high-dose supplementation with vitamins C and E, beta carotene, and zinc for age-related macular degeneration and vision loss: AREDS report Archives of Ophthalmology. (2001). , 119(8), 1417-1436.

[86] Moriarty-craige, S. E, Adkison, J, Lynn, M, Gensler, G, Bressler, S, & Jones, D. P. Sternberg P Jr. Antioxidant supplements prevent oxidation of cysteine/cystine redox in patients with age-related macular degeneration. Am J Ophthalmol. (2005). , 140, 1020-1026.

[87] Jakobsdottir, J, Conley, Y. P, Weeks, D. E, Mah, T. S, Ferrell, R. E, & Gorin, M. B. Susceptibility genes for age-related maculopathy on chromosome 10q26. Am J of Human Genetics. (2005). , 77(3), 389-407.

[88] Rivera, A, Fisher, S. A, Fritsche, L. G, Keilhauer, C. N, Lichtner, P, Meitinger, T, & Weber, B. H. Hypothetical LOC387715 is a second major susceptibility gene for age-related macular degeneration, contributing independently of complement factor H to disease risk. Human Molecular Genetics. (2005). , 14(21), 3227-3236.

[89] Schmidt, S, Hauser, M. A, Scott, W. K, Postel, E. A, Agarwal, A, Gallins, P, Wong, F, Chen, Y. S, Spencer, K, Schnetz-boutaud, N, Haines, J. L, & Pericak-vance, M. A. Cigarette smoking strongly modifies the association of LOC387715 and age-related macular degeneration. Am J of Human Genetics. (2006). , 78(5), 852-864.

[90] Kanda, A, Chen, W, Othman, M, Branham, K. E, Brooks, M, Khanna, R, He, S, Lyons, R, Abecasis, G. R, & Swaroop, A. A variant of mitochondrial protein LOC387715/ARMS2, not HTRA1, is strongly associated with age-related macular degeneration. Proceedings of the National Academy of Sciences USA, (2007). , 41, 16227-16232.

[91] Gu, X, Meer, S. G, Miyagi, M, Rayborn, M. E, Hollyfield, J. G, Crabb, J. W, & Salomon, R. G. Carboxyethylpyrrole protein adducts and autoantibodies, biomarkers for age-related macular degeneration. Jl of Biol Chem. (2003). , 43, 42027-42035.

[92] SunML; Finnemann,SC; Febbraio, M; Shan, L; Annangudi, SP; Podrez, EA; Hoppe, G; Darrow, R; Organisciak, DT; Salomon, RG; Silverstein, RL; Hazen, S. Light-induced oxidation of photoreceptor outer segment phospholipids generates ligands for CD36-mediated phagocytosis by retinal pigment epithelium: A potential mechanism for modulating outer segment phagocytosis under oxidant stress conditions. J Biol Chem. (2006). , 281(7), 4222-4230.

[93] Schutt, F, Bergmann, M, Holz, F. G, & Kopitz, J. Proteins modified by malondialdehyde, 4-hydroxynonenal, or advanced glycation end products in lipofuscin of human retinal pigment epithelium. Invest Ophthalmol Vis Sci. (2003). , 44(8), 3663-3668.

[94] Schutt, F, Ueberle, B, Schnölzer, M, Holz, F. G, & Kopitz, J. Proteome analysis of lipofuscin in human retinal pigment epithelial cells. FEBS Letters. (2002). , 528, 217-221.

[95] Crabb, J. W, Miyagi, M, Gu, X, Shadrach, K, West, K. A, Sakaguchi, H, Kamei, M, Hasan, A, Yan, L, Rayborn, M. E, Salomon, R. G, & Hollyfield, J. G. Drusen proteome analysis: An approach to the etiology of age-related macular degeneration. Proc Natl Acad Sci U SA. (2002). , 99(23), 14682-14687.

[96] Farboud, B, Aotaki-keen, A, Miyata, T, Hjelmeland, L. M, & Handa, J. T. Development of a polyclonal antibody with broad epitope specificity for advanced glycation endproducts and localization of these epitopes in Bruch's membrane of the aging eye. Molecular Vision. (1999).

[97] Biswas, S. K, & Rahman, I. Environmental toxicity, redox signaling and lung inflammation: The role of glutathione. Molecular Aspects of Medicine. (2009).

[98] Edwards, A. O, & Ritter, R. rd, Abel KJ, Manning A, Panhuysen C, Farrer LA.Complement factor H polymorphism and age-related macular degeneration. Science. (2005)., 308(5720), 421-424.

[99] Zareparsi, S, Branham, K. E, Li, M, Shah, S, Klein, R. J, Ott, J, Hoh, J, Abecasis, G. R, & Swaroop, A. Strong association of the Y402H variant in complement factor H at 1q32 with susceptibility to age-related macular degeneration. Am J of Hum Gen. (2005)., 77(1), 149-153.

[100] Ding, X, Patel, M, & Chan, C. C. Molecular pathology of age-related macular degeneration. Prog Retin Eye Res. (2009)., 28(1), 1-18.

[101] Chen, H, Liu, B, Lukas, T. J, & Neufeld, A. H. The aged retinal pigment epithelium/choroid: a potential substratum for the pathogenesis of age-related macular degeneration. PLoS One, (2008). Jun 4;3(6):e2339.

[102] Scott, W. K, Schmidt, S, Hauser, M. A, Gallins, P, Schnetz-boutaud, N, Spencer, K. L, Gilbert, J. R, Agarwal, A, & Postel, E. A. Haines Jl, Pericak-Vance MA. Independent effects of complement factor H Y402H polymorphism and cigarette smoking on risk of age-related macular degeneration. Ophthalmology. (2007)., 114, 1151-1156.

[103] Schmidt, S, Haines, J. L, Postel, E. A, & Agarwal, A. Kwan SY; Gilbert JR, Pericak-Vance MA, Scott WK. Joint effects of smoking history and APOE genotypes in age-related macular degeneration. Mol Vis, (2005)., 11, 941-949.

[104] Bertram, K. M, Baglole, C. J, Phipps, R. P, & Libby, R. T. Molecular regulation of cigarette smoke induced-oxidative stress in human retinal pigment epithelial cells: implications for age-related macular degeneration. Am J Physiol Cell Physiol. (2009). C , 1200-1210.

[105] Wang, A. L, Lukas, T. J, Yuan, M, Du, N, Handa, J. T, & Neufeld, A. H. Changes in retinal pigment epithelium related to cigarette smoke: possible relevance to smoking as a risk factor for age-related macular degeneration. PLoS One. (2009). e5304.

[106] Hollyfield, J. G, Bonilha, V. L, Rayborn, M. E, Yang, X, Shadrach, K. G, Lu, L, Ugret, R. L, Salomon, R. G, & Perez, V. L. Oxidative damage-induced inflammation initiates age related macular degeneration. Nat. Med. (2008).

[107] Mahapatra, S. K, Das, S, Bhattacharjee, S, Gautam, N, Majumdar, S, & Roy, S. Toxicol Mech Methods. (2009)., 19(2), 100-108.

[108] Maritz, G. S. Nicotine and lung development. Birth Defects Res C Embryo Today. (2008)., 84(1), 45-53.

[109] Das, S, Neogy, S, Gautan, N, & Roy, S. In vitro nicotine induced superoxide mediated DNA fragmentation in lymphocytes: protective role of Andrographis paniculata Nees. Toxicology in Vitro. (2009). , 23, 909-998.

[110] Vassallo, R, Kroening, P. R, Parambil, J, & Kita, H. Nicotine and cigarette smoke constituents induce-immune-modulatory and pro-inflammatory dendritic cell responses. Mol Immunol. (2008). , 45(12), 3321-3329.

[111] Pestana, I. A, Vazquez-padron, R. I, Aitouche, A, & Pham, S. M. Nicotine and PDGF-receptor function are essential for nicotine-stimulated mitogenesis in human vascular smooth muscle cells. J Cell Biochem. (2005). , 965, 986-995.

[112] Suner, I, Espinosa-heidmann, D. G, Marin-castano, M. E, & Hernandez, E. Pereira-Simon S Cousins SW. Nicotine increase size and severity of experimental choroidal neovascularization. Invest. Ophthalmol. Vis. Sci. (2004). , 451, 311-317.

[113] Villablanca, A. C. Nicotine stimulates DNA synthesis and proliferation in vascular endothelial cell in vitro. J. Appl. Physiol. (1998). , 846, 2086-2098.

[114] Kiuchi, K, Matsuoka, M, & Wu, J. C. Lima e Silva R, Kengatharan M, Verghese M, Ueno S, Yokoi K, Khu NH, Cooke JP, Campochiaro PA. Mecamylamine suppresses basal and nicotine-stimulated choroidal neovascularization. Invest Ophthalmol Vis Sci. (2008). , 49(4), 1705-11.

[115] KandaY; Watanabe, Y. Nicotine-induced vascular endothelial growth factor release via the EGFR-ERK pathway in rat vascular smooth muscle cells. Life Sci, (2007). , 8015, 1409-1414.

[116] Ishibashi, T, Hata, Y, Yosikawa, H, Nakagawa, K, Sueishi, K, & Inomata, H. Expression of vascular endothelial growth factor in experimental choroidal neovascularization. Graefes Arch Clin Exp Ophthalmol. (1997). , 2353, 159-167.

[117] Kliffen, M, Sharma, H. S, Mooy, C. M, Kerkvliet, S, & De Jong, P. T. Increased expression of angiogenic growth factor in age-related maculopathy. Br J Ophthalmology. (1997). , 812, 154-162.

[118] Kvanta, A. Ocular angiogenesis: the role of growth factors. Acta Ophthalmol. (2006). , 843, 282-288.

[119] Hyman, L, & Neborsky, R. Risk factors for age-related macular degeneration: an update Current Opinion in Ophthalmology. (2002). , 13(3), 171-175.

[120] Vingerling, J. R, Klaver, C. C, & Hofman, A. Epidemiology of age-related maculopathy. Epidemiol.Rev. (1995). , 17, 347-360.

[121] Bilato, C, & Crow, M. T. Atherosclerosis and the vascular biology of aging. Aging (Milano), (1996). , 8, 221-234.

[122] Hariri, R. J, Alonso, D. R, & Hajjar, D. P. Aging and arteriosclerosis. I. Development of myointimal hyperplasia after endothelial injury. J Exp.Med, (1986). , 164, 1171-1178.

[123] Spagnoli, L. G, Sambuy, Y, & Palmieri, G. Age-related modulation of vascular smooth muscle cells proliferation following arterial wall damage. Artery, (1985). , 13, 187-198.

[124] Jonas, J. B, Hayreh, S. S, & Martus, P. Influence of arterial hypertension and diet-induced atherosclerosis on macular drusen. Graefe's archive for clinical and experimental ophthalmology = Albrecht von Graefes Archiv fur klinische und experimentelle Ophthalmologie. (2003). , 241(2), 125-134.

[125] Olea, J. L, & Tuñón, J. Patients with neovascular age-related macular degeneration in Spain display a high cardiovascular risk. Eur J Ophthalmol. (2012). , 22(3), 404-11.

[126] Hogg, R. E, Woodside, J. V, Gilchrist, S. E, Graydon, R, Fletcher, A. E, Chan, W, Knox, A, Cartmill, B, & Chakravarthy, U. Cardiovascular disease and hypertension are strong risk factors for choroidal neovascularization. Ophthalmology. (2008). , 115(6), 1046-1052.

[127] Thapa, R, Paudyal, G, Shrestha, M. K, Gurung, R, & Ruit, S. Age-related macular degeneration in Nepal. Kathmandu Univ Med J (KUMJ). (2011). , 9(35), 165-9.

[128] Hogg, R. E, Mckay, G. J, Hughes, A. E, Muldrew, K. A, & Chakravarthy, U. GENOTYPE-PHENOTYPE ASSOCIATIONS IN NEOVASCULAR AGE-RELATED MACULAR DEGENERATION. Retina. (2012). Apr 5. (Epub ahead of print).

[129] Ruiz-OrtegaM; Ruperez, M; Esteban, V. Molecular Mechanisms of Angiotensin II-induced Vascular Injury. Curr Hypertens.Rep, (2003). , 5, 73-79.

[130] Taylor, W. R. Hypertensive vascular disease and inflammation: mechanical and humoral mechanisms. Curr Hypertens.Rep, (1999). , 1, 96-101.

[131] DoreyCK; Wu, G; Ebenstein, D. Cell loss in the aging retina. Relationship to lipofuscin accumulation and macular degeneration. Invest Ophthalmol Vis Sci,(1989). , 30, 1691-1699.

[132] Rong, P, Wilkinson-berka, J. L, & Skinner, S. L. Control of renin secretion from adrenal gland in transgenic Ren-2 and normal rats. Mol Cell Endocrinol. (2001). , 173, 203-212.

[133] Wilkinson-berka, J. L, Kelly, D. J, Rong, P, Campbell, D. J, & Skinner, S. L. Characterisation of a thymic renin-angiotensin system in the transgenic m(Ren-2)27 rat. Mol Cell Endocrinol. (2002). , 194, 201-209.

[134] Berka, J. L, Stubbs, A. J, & Wang, D. Z. DiNicolantonio R, Alcorn D, Campbell DJ, Skinner SL (1995). Renin-containing Muller cells of the retina display endocrine features. Invest Ophthalmol Vis Sci. (1995). , 36, 1450-1458.

[135] Sarlos, S, Rizkalla, B, Moravski, C. J, Cao, Z, Cooper, M. E, & Wilkinson-berka, J. L. Retinal angiogenesis is mediated by an interaction between the angiotensin type 2 receptor, VEGF, and angiopoietin. Am J Pathol. (2003). , 163, 879-887.

[136] Senanayake, P, Drazba, J, Shadrach, K, Milsted, A, Rungger-brandle, E, Nishiyama, K, Miura, S, Karnik, S, Sears, J. E, Hollyfield, J. G, & Angiotensin, I. I. and its receptor subtypes in the human retina. Invest Ophthalmol Vis Sci. (2007). , 48, 3301-3311.

[137] Downie, L. E, Vessey, K, Miller, A, Ward, M. M, Pianta, M. J, Vingrys, A. J, Wilkinson-berka, J. L, & Fletcher, E. L. Neuronal and glial cell expression of angiotensin II type 1 (AT1) and type 2 (AT2) receptors in the rat retina. Neuroscience. (2009). , 161, 195-213.

[138] Milenkovic, V. M, Brockmann, M, Meyer, C, Desch, M, Schweda, F, Kurtz, A, Todorov, V, & Strauss, O. Regulation of the renin expression in the retinal pigment epithelium by systemic stimuli. Am J Physiol Renal Physiol. (2010). FF403., 396.

[139] Fletcher, E. L, Phipps, J. A, Ward, M. M, Vessey, K. A, & Wilkinson-berka, J. L. The renin-angiotensin system in retinal health and disease: Its influence on neurons, glia and the vasculature. Prog Retin Eye Res. (2010). , 29, 284-311.

[140] Wagner, J. Jan Danser AH, Derkx FH, de Jong TV, Paul M, Mullins JJ, Schalekamp MA, Ganten D. Demonstration of renin mRNA, angiotensinogen mRNA, and angiotensin convertingenzyme mRNA expression in the human eye: evidence for an intraocular renin-angiotensin system.Br J Ophthalmol. (1996). , 80, 159-163.

[141] Jacobi, P. C, Osswald, H, Jurklies, B, & Zrenner, E. Neuromodulatory effects of the reninangiotensin system on the cat electroretinogram. Invest Ophthalmol Vis Sci. (1994). , 35, 973-980.

[142] Jurklies, B, Eckstein, A, Jacobi, P, Kohler, K, Risler, T, & Zrenner, E. The renin-angiotensin system--a possible neuromodulator in the human retina? Ger J Ophthalmol. (1995). , 4, 144-150.

[143] Danser, A. H, Derkx, F. H, Admiraal, P. J, Deinum, J, De Jong, P. T, & Schalekamp, M. A. (1994). Angiotensin levels in the eye. Invest Ophthalmol Vis Sci , 35, 1008-1018.

[144] Wilkinson-berka, J. L, Tan, G, Jaworski, K, & Ninkovic, S. Valsartan but not atenolol improves vascular pathology in diabetic Ren-2 rat retina. Am J Hypertens. (2007). , 20, 423-430.

[145] Mauer, M, Zinman, B, Gardiner, R, Suissa, S, Sinaiko, A, Strand, T, Drummond, K, Donnelly, S, Goodyer, P, Gubler, M. C, & Klein, R. Renal and retinal effects of enalapril and losartan in type 1 diabetes. N Engl J Med. (2009). , 361, 40-51.

[146] Moravski, C. J, Kelly, D. J, Cooper, M. E, Gilbert, R. E, Bertram, J. F, Shahinfar, S, Skinner, S. L, & Wilkinson-berka, J. L. Retinal neovascularization is prevented by blockade of the renin-angiotensin system. Hypertension. (2000). , 36, 1099-1104.

[147] Nagai, N, Noda, K, Urano, T, Kubota, Y, Shinoda, H, Koto, T, Shinoda, K, Inoue, M, Shiomi, T, Ikeda, E, Tsubota, K, Suda, T, Oike, Y, & Ishida, S. Selective suppression of pathologic, but not physiologic, retinal neovascularization by blocking the angiotensin II type 1 receptor. Invest Ophthalmol Vis Sci. (2005). , 46, 1078-1084.

[148] Downie, L. E, Pianta, M. J, Vingrys, A. J, Wilkinson-berka, J. L, & Fletcher, E. L. AT1 receptor inhibition prevents astrocyte degeneration and restores vascular growth in oxygen-induced retinopathy. Glia. (2008). , 56, 1076-1090.

[149] Nagai, N, Oike, Y, Izumi-nagai, K, Koto, T, Satofuka, S, Shinoda, H, Noda, K, Ozawa, Y, Inoue, M, Tsubota, K, & Ishida, S. Suppression of choroidal neovascularization by inhibiting angiotensinconverting enzyme: minimal role of bradykinin. Invest Ophthalmol Vis Sci. (2007). , 48, 2321-2326.

[150] Jin, G. F, & Hurst, J. S. Godley BF cultured human retinal pigment epithelial cells. Curr Eye Res. (2001). , 22, 165-173.

[151] Yamada, H, Yamada, E, Hackett, S. F, Ozaki, H, Okamoto, N, & Campochiaro, P. A. Hyperoxia causes decreased expression of vascular endothelial growth factor and endothelial cell apoptosis in adult retina. J Cell Physiol. (1999). , 179, 149-156.

[152] Hecquet, C, Lefevre, G, Valtink, M, Engelmann, K, & Mascarelli, F. Activation and role of MAP kinase-dependent pathways in retinal pigment epithelium cells: JNK1, kinase, and cell death. Invest Ophthalmol Vis Sci. (2003). , 38.

[153] Dunaief, J. L, Dentchev, T, Ying, G. S, & Milam, A. H. The role of apoptosis in age-related macular degeneration. Arch Ophthalmol. (2002). , 120, 1435-1442.

[154] Florence, T. M. The role of free radicals in disease. Australian and New Zealand Journal of Ophthalmology. (1995). , 23(1), 3-7.

[155] Machlin, L. J, & Bendich, A. Free radical tissue damage: protective role of antioxidant nutrients The FASEB journal : official publication of the Federation of American Societies for Experimental Biology. (1987). , 1(6), 441-445.

[156] Stohs, S. J. The role of free radicals in toxicity and disease. Journal of Basic and Clinical Physiology and Pharmacology. (1995).

[157] Beatty, S, Koh, H, Phil, M, Henson, D, & Boulton, M. The role of oxidative stress in the pathogenesis of age-related macular degeneration. Survey of Ophthalmology. (2000). , 45(2), 115-134.

[158] Wilhelm, J. Metabolic aspects of membrane lipid peroxidation. Acta Universitatis Carolinae. Medica. Monographia. (1990). , 137, 1-53.

[159] Blokhina, O, Virolainen, E, & Fagerstedt, K. V. Antioxidants, oxidative damage and oxygen deprivation stress: a review. Annals of Botany. (2003). Spec (179-194), 179-194.

[160] Iwai, K. An ubiquitin ligase recognizing a protein oxidized by iron: implications for the turnover of oxidatively damaged proteins. Journal of Biochemistry. (2003). , 134(2), 175-182.

[161] Hugel, B. Martinez mC, Kunzelmann C, Freyssinet JM. Membrane microparticles: two sides of the coin. Physiology. (2005). , 20, 22-27.

[162] Nomura, S, Ozaki, Y, & Ikeda, Y. Function and role of microparticles in various clinical setting. Thromb Res. (2008). , 123, 8-23.

[163] Mostefai, H. A, Andriantsitohaina, R, & Martinez, M. C. Plasma membrane microparticles in angiogenesis: role in ischemic diseases and cancer. Physiol Res. (2008). , 57, 311-320.

[164] Van Wijk, D, & Simons, M. Microparticles in cardiovascular diseases. Cardiovasc Res. (2003). , 59, 1121-1132.

[165] Negi, A, & Marmor, M. F. Experimental serous retinal detachment and focal pigment epithelial damage. Arch Ophthalmol. (1984). , 102(3), 445-9.

[166] Van Der Schaft, T. L, De Bruijn, B. C, & Mooy, G. M. Ketelaars DAM, Jong PTVM. Is basal laminar deposit unique for age-related macular degeneration?. Arch Ophthalmol (1991). , 109, 420-425.

[167] Burns, R. Feeney Burns L. Clinico-morphologic correlations of drusen of Bruch's membrane. Trans Am Ophthalmol Soc. (1980). , 78, 206-225.

[168] Gerthoffer, W. T, & Gunst, S. J. Invited review: focal adhesion and small heat shock proteins in the regulation of actin remodeling and contractility in smooth muscle. J Appl Physiol. (2001). , 91, 963-972.

[169] Zhu, Z. R, Goodnight, R, Nishimura, T, Sorgente, N, Ogden, T. E, & Ryan, S. J. Experimental changes resembling the pathology of drusen in Bruch's membrane in the rabbit. Curr Eye Res.(1988). , 7, 581-592.

[170] Malorni, W, Iosi, F, Mirabelli, F, & Bellomo, G. Cytoskeleton as a target in menadione-induced oxidative stress in cultured mammalian cells: alterations underlying surface bleb formation. Chem Biol Interact. (1991). , 80, 217-236.

[171] Marin-castaño, M. E, Csaky, K. G, & Cousins, S. W. Nonlethal oxidant injury to human retinal pigment epithelium cells causes cell membrane blebbing but decreased MMP-2 activity. Invest Ophthalmol Vis Sci. (2005). , 46(9), 3331-3340.

[172] Stein, J. M, & Luzio, J. P. complement attack on human neutrophils. The sorting of endogenous plasma-membrane proteins and lipids into shed vesicles. Biochem. J. (1991). , 274, 381-386.

[173] Combes, V, Simon, A. C, Grau, G. E, Arnoux, D, Camoin, L, Sabatier, F, Mutin, M, Sanmarco, M, Sampol, J, & Dignat-george, F. In vitro generation of endothelial micro-

particles and possible prothrombotic activity in patients with lupus anticoagulant. J. Clin. Investig. (1999). , 104, 93-102.

[174] Sims, P. J, Faioni, E. M, Wiedmer, T, & Shattil, S. J. Complement proteins C5b-9 cause release of membrane vesicles from the platelet surface that are enriched in the membrane receptor for coagulation factor Va and express prothrombinase activity. J. Biol. Chem. (1988). , 263, 18205-18212.

[175] Iida, K, Whitlow, M. B, & Nussenzweig, V. Membrane vesiculation protects erythrocytes from destruction by complement. J. Immunol. (1991). , 147, 2638-2642.

[176] Pascual, M, Steiger, G, Sadallah, S, Paccaud, J. P, Carpentier, J. L, James, R, & Schifferli, J. A. Identification of membrane-bound CR1 (CD35) in human urine: evidence for its release by glomerular podocytes. J. Exp. Med. (1994). , 179, 889-899.

[177] Satta, N, Toti, F, Feugeas, O, Bohbot, A, Dachary-prigent, J, Eschwège, V, Hedman, H, & Freyssinet, J. M. Monocyte vesiculation is a possible mechanism for dissemination of membrane-associated procoagulant activities and adhesion molecules after stimulation by lipopolysaccharide. J. Immunol. (1994). , 153, 3245-3255.

[178] Bütikofer, P. Kuypers, Xu CM, Chiu DT, Lubin B. Enrichment of two glycosyl-phosphatidylinositol-anchored proteins, acetylcholinesterase and decay accelerating factor, in vesicles released from human red blood cells. Blood; , 74, 1481-1485.

[179] Alcazar, O, Collier, T. S, Cousins, S. W, Bhattacharya, S. K, Muddiman, D. C, & Marin-castano, M. E. Proteomics Characterization of Cell Membrane Blebs in Human Retinal Pigment Epithelium Cells. Mol Cell Proteomics. (2009). , 8(10), 2201-2211.

[180] Dalle-donne, I, Rossi, R, & Milzani, A. Di Simplicio P, Colombo R. The actin cytoskeleton response to oxidants: from small heat shock protein phosphorylation to changes in the redox state of actin itself. Free Radic Biol Med. (2001). , 31(12), 1624-1632.

[181] Lanzetti, L. Di Fiore PP, Scita G. Pathways linking endocytosis and actin cytoskeleton in mammalian cells. Exp Cell Res. (2001). , 271(1), 45-56.

[182] Taunton, J. Actin filament nucleation by endosomes, lysosomes and secretory vesicles. Curr Opin Cell Biol. (2001). , 13(1), 85-91.

[183] Rao, A, & Craig, A. M. Signaling between the actin cytoskeleton and the postsynaptic density of dendritic spines. Hippocampus. (2000). , 10(5), 527-541.

[184] Kaibuchi, K, Kuroda, S, & Amano, M. Regulation of the cytoskeleton and cell adhesion by the Rho family GTPases in mammalian cells. Annu Rev Biochem. (1999). , 68, 459-486.

[185] Valentijn, K, Valentijn, J. A, & Jamieson, J. D. Role of actin in regulated exocytosis and compensatory membrane retrieval: insights from an old acquaintance. Biochem Biophys Res Commun.(1999). , 266(3), 652-661.

[186] Downey, G. P. Mechanisms of leukocyte motility and chemotaxis. Curr Opin Immunol. (1994)., 6(1), 113-124.

[187] Hirokawa, N. Axonal transport and the cytoskeleton. Curr Opin Neurobiol. (1993)., 3(5), 724-731.

[188] Weed, S. A, & Parsons, J. T. Cortactin: coupling membrane dynamics to cortical actin assembly. Oncogene. (2001)., 20(44), 6418-6434.

[189] Milzani, A. DalleDonne I, Colombo R, Rodriguez OC. Prolonged oxidative stress on actin. Arch Biochem Biophys. (1997)., 339(2), 267-274.

[190] Huot, J, Houle, F, Rousseau, S, Deschesnes, R. G, Shah, G. M, Landry, J, & Sapk, p. dependent F-actin reorganization regulates early membrane blebbing during stress-induced apoptosis. J Cell Biol. (1998)., 143(5), 1361-1373.

[191] ConcannonCG; Gorman, AM; Samali, A. On the role of Hsp27 in regulating apoptosis. Apoptosis. (2003)., 8(1), 61-70.

[192] Delogu, G, Signore, M, Mechelli, A, & Famularo, G. Heat shock proteins and their role in heart injury. Curr Opin Crit Care. (2002)., 8(5), 411-416.

[193] Ganea, E. Chaperone-like activity of alpha-crystallin and other small heat shock proteins. Curr Protein Pept Sci. (2001)., 2(3), 205-225.

[194] De Lanerolle, P, & Cole, A. B. Cytoskeletal proteins and gene regulation: form, function, and signal transduction in the nucleus. Sci STKE. (2002). E30.

[195] Landry, J, & Huot, J. Modulation of actin dynamics during stress and physiological stimulation by a signaling pathway involving MAP kinase and heat-shock protein 27. Biochem Cell Biol. (1995)., 38.

[196] Stokoe, D, Engel, K, Campbell, D. G, Cohen, P, & Gaestel, M. Identification of MAPKAP kinase 2 as a major enzyme responsible for the phosphorylation of the small mammalian heat shock proteins. FEBS Lett. (1992)., 313(3), 307-313.

[197] Gerthoffer, W. T, & Gunst, S. J. Invited review: focal adhesion and small heat shock proteins in the regulation of actin remodeling and contractility in smooth muscle. J Appl Physiol. (2001)., 91, 963-972.

[198] Huot, J, Houle, F, Marceau, F, & Landry, J. Oxidative stress-induced actin reorganization mediated by the mitogen-activated protein kinase/heat shock protein 27 pathway in vascular endothelial cells. Circ Res. (1997)., 38.

[199] Lavoie, J. N, Lambert, H, Hickey, E, Weber, L. A, & Landry, J. Modulation of cellular thermoresistance and actin filament stability accompanies phosphorylation-induced changes in the oligomeric structure of heat shock protein 27. Mol Cell Biol. (1995)., 15, 505-516.

[200] GuayJ; Lambert, H; Gingras-Breton, G; Lavoie, JN; Huot, J; Landry, J. Regulation of actinfilament dynamics by map kinase-mediated phosphorylation of heat shock protein 27. J Cell Sci. (1997). , 38.

[201] ClerkA; Michael, A; Sugden, PH. Stimulation of multiple mitogen-activated protein kinase sub-families by oxidative stress and phosphorylation of the small heat shock protein, HSP25/27, in neonatal ventricular myocytes. Biochem J. (1998). , 333(3), 581-589.

[202] GusevNB; Bogatcheva, NV; Marston, SB. Structure and properties of small heat shock proteins (sHsp) and their interaction with cytoskeleton proteins. Biochemistry (Mosc). (2002). , 67, 511-519.

[203] Shi, B, Han, B, Schwab, I. R, & Isseroff, R. R. UVB irradiation-induced changes in the 27-kd heat shock protein (HSP27) in human corneal epithelial cells. Cornea. (2006). , 25, 948-955.

[204] Decanini, A, Nordgaard, C. L, Feng, X, Ferrington, D. A, & Olsen, T. W. Changes in select redox proteins of the retinal pigment epithelium in age-related macular degeneration. Am J Ophthalmol. (2007). , 143, 607-615.

[205] Pons, M, Cousins, S. W, Csaky, K. G, Striker, G, & Marin-castaño, M. E. Cigarette smoke-related hydroquinone induces filamentous actin reorganization and heat shock protein 27 phosphorylation through and extracellular signal-regulated kinase 1/2 in retinal pigment epithelium: implications for age-related macular degeneration. Am J Pathol. (2010). , 38.

[206] Strunnikova, N, Baffi, J, Gonzalez, A, Silk, W, Cousins, S. W, & Csaky, K. G. Regulated heat shock protein 27 expression in human retinal pigment epithelium. Invest Ophthalmol Vis Sci. (2001). , 42, 2130-2138.

[207] Cuenda, A, Rouse, J, Doza, Y. N, Meier, R, Cohen, P, Gallagher, T. F, Young, P. R, Lee, J. C, & Is, S. B. a specific inhibitor of a MAP kinase homologue which is stimulated by cellular stresses and interleukin-1. FEBS Lett. (1995). , 364, 229-233.

[208] Huot, J, Lambert, H, Lavoie, J. N, Guimond, A, Houle, F, & Landry, J. Characterization of 45-kDa/54-kDa HSP27 kinase, a stress-sensitive kinase which may activate the phosphorylationdependent protective function of mammalian 27-kDa heat-shock protein HSP27. Eur J Biochem. (1995). , 227, 416-427.

[209] Cairns, J, Qin, S, Philp, R, Tan, Y. H, & Guy, G. R. Dephosphorylation of the small heat shock protein Hsp27 in vivo by protein phosphatase 2A. J Biol Chem, (1994). , 269, 9176-9183.

[210] Kostenko, S, & Moens, U. Heat shock protein 27 phosphorylation: kinases, phosphatases,functions and pathology. Cell Mol Life Sci. (2009). , 66, 3289-3307.

[211] Garg, T. K, & Chang, J. Y. Oxidative stress causes ERK phosphorylation and cell death in cultured retinal pigment epithelium: prevention of cell death by AG126 and 15-deoxy-delta PGJ2. BMC Ophthalmol. (2003). , 12, 14.

[212] Chiang, J, & Kowada, M. Ames III A, Wright RL, Majino G. Cerebral isquenia III. Vascular changes. Am. J. Path. (1968). , 52, 437-447.

[213] Feig, L. A. Ral-GTPases: approaching their 15 minutes of fame. Trends Cell Biol. (2003). , 13, 419-425.

[214] Charras, G. T. A short history of blebbing. J Microsc. (2008). , 231, 466-478.

[215] Takai, Y, Sasaki, T, & Matozaki, T. Small GTP-binding proteins. Physiol Rev. (2001). , 81, 153-208.

[216] Albright, C. F, Giddings, B. W, Liu, J, Vito, M, & Weinberg, R. A. Characterization of a guanine nucleotide dissociation stimulator for a ras-related GTPase. EMBO J. (1993). , 12, 339-347.

[217] Hofer, F, Fields, S, Schneider, C, & Martin, G. S. Activated Ras interacts with the Ral guanine nucleotide dissociation stimulator. Proc Natl Acad Sci USA. (1994). , 91, 11089-11093.

[218] Kikuchi, A, & Williams, L. T. Regulation of interaction of ras with RalGDS and Raf-1 by cyclic AMP-dependent protein kinase. J Biol Chem. (1996). , 21.

[219] Matsubara, K, Kishida, S, Matsuura, Y, Kitayama, H, Noda, M, & Kikuchi, A. Plasma membrane recruitment of RalGDS is critical for Ras-dependent Ral activation. Oncogene. (1999). , 18, 1303-1312.

[220] Wolthuis, R. M, & Bos, J. L. Ras caught in another affair: the exchange factors for Ral. Curr Opin Genet Dev. (1999). , 9, 112-117.

[221] Barnes, W. G, Reiter, E, Violin, J. D, Ren, X. R, Milligan, G, & Lefkowitz, R. J. beta-Arrestin 1 and Galphaq/11 coordinately activate RhoA and stress fiber formation following receptor stimulation. J Biol Chem. (2005). , 280, 8041-8050.

[222] Matrougui, K, Tankó, L. B, Loufrani, L, Gorny, D, Levy, B. I, Tedgui, A, & Henrion, D. Involvement of Rho-kinase and the actin filament network in angiotensin II-induced contraction and extracellular signal-regulated kinase activity in intact rat mesenteric resistance arteries. Arterioscler Thromb Vasc Biol. (2001). , 21, 1288-1293.

[223] Lammers, M, Meyer, S, Kühlmann, D, & Wittinghofer, A. Specificity of interactions between mDia isoforms and Rho proteins. J Biol Chem. (2008). , 283, 35236-35246.

[224] Krebs, A, Rothkegel, M, Klar, M, & Jockusch, B. M. Characterization of functional domains of mDia1, a link between the small GTPase Rho and the actin cytoskeleton. J Cell Sci. (2001). , 114, 3663-3672.

[225] Godin, C. M, & Ferguson, S. S. The angiotensin II type 1 receptor induces membrane blebbing by coupling to Rho A, Rho kinase, and myosin light chain kinase. Mol Pharmacol. (2010).

[226] Min Kim JUehara Y, Ja Choi Y, Mi Ha Y, Hyeok, Ye, B, Pal Yu B, Young Chung H. Mecahnism of attenuation of pro-inflammatory Ang II-induced NF-kB activation by genistein in the kidneys of male rats during aging. Biogerontology. (2011). DOIs10522-011-9345-4).

[227] Aumailley, M, & Gayraud, B. Structure and biological activity of the extracellular matrix. J Mol Med. (1998). , 76, 253-265.

[228] Kugler, A. Matrix metalloproteinases and their inhibitors. Anticancer Res. (1999). , 19, 1589-1592.

[229] Jacot, T. A, Striker, G. E, & Stetler-stevenson, M. Mesangial cells from transgenic mice with progressive glomerulosclerosis exhibit stable, phenotypic changes including undetectable MMP-9 and increased type IV collagen. Lab Invest. (1996). , 75, 791-799.

[230] Peten, E. P, Garcia-perez, A, & Terada, Y. Age-related changes in alpha and alpha 2-chain type IV collagen mRNAs in adult mouse glomeruli: competitive PCR. Am J Physiol. (1992). F951-F957., 1.

[231] Belkhiri, A, Richards, C, & Whaley, M. Increased expression of activated matrix metalloproteinase-2 by human endothelial cells after sublethal H2O2 exposure. Lab Inves. (1997). , 77, 533-539.

[232] Alcazar, O, Cousins, S. W, & Marin-castaño, M. E. MMP-14 and TIMP-2 overexpression protects against hydroquinone-induced oxidant injury in RPE: implications for extracellular matrix turnover. Invest Ophthalmol Vis Sci. (2007). , 48(12), 5662-70.

[233] Wiesner, C, Faix, J, Himmel, M, Bentzien, F, Linder, S, & Kif, B. and KIF3A/KIF3B kinesins drive MT1-MMP surface exposure, CD44 shedding, and extracellular matrix degradation in primary macrophages. Blood. (2010). , 116(9), 1559-69.

[234] Zhang, C, Baffi, J, Cousins, S. W, & Csaky, K. G. Oxidant-induced cell death in retinal pigment epithelium cells mediated through the release of apoptosis-inducing factor. J Cell Sci. (2003). , 116(10), 1915-1923.

[235] Cousins, S. W, Marin-castano, M. E, Espinosa-heidmann, D. G, Alexandridou, A, Striker, L, & Elliot, S. Female gender, estrogen loss, and Sub-RPE deposit formation in aged mice. Invest Ophthalmol Vis Sci. (2003). , 44(3), 1221-1229.

[236] Fossum, S, Mallett, S, & Barclay, A. N. The MRC OX-47 antigen is a member of the immunoglobulin superfamily with an unusual transmembrane sequence. Eur J Immunol. (1991). , 21, 671-679.

[237] Miyauchi, T, Masuzawa, Y, & Muramatsu, T. The basigin group of the immunoglobulin superfamily: complete conservation of a segment in and around transmem-

brane domains of human and mouse basigin and chicken HT7 antigen. J Biochem. (1991)., 110, 770-774.

[238] Kasinrerk, W, Fiebiger, E, Stefanová, I, Baumruker, T, Knapp, W, & Stockinger, H. Human leukocyte activation antigen M6, a member of the Ig superfamily, is the species homologue of rat OX-47, mouse basigin, and chicken HT7 molecule. J Immunol. (1992)., 149, 847-854.

[239] Kasinrerk, W, Tokrasinwit, N, & Phunpae, P. CD147 monoclonal antibodies induce homotypic cell aggregation of monocytic cell line U937 via LFA-1/ICAM-1 pathway. Immunology. (1999)., 96, 184-192.

[240] Biswas, C, Zhang, Y, Decastro, R, Guo, H, Nakamura, T, Kataoka, H, & Nabeshima, K. The human tumor cell-derived collagenase stimulatory factor (renamed EMMPRIN) is a member of the immunoglobulin superfamily. Cancer Res. (1995). , 55, 434-439.

[241] Biswas, C. Tumor cell stimulation of collagenase production by fibroblasts. Biochem Biophys Res Commun. (1982)., 109, 1026-1034.

[242] Kataoka, H, Decastro, R, Zucker, S, & Biswas, C. Tumor cell-derived collagenase-stimulatory factor increases expression of interstitial collagenase, stromelysin, and 72-kDa gelatinase. Cancer Res. (1993)., 53, 3154-3148.

[243] Guo, H, Zucker, S, Gordon, M. K, Toole, B. P, & Biswas, C. Stimulation of matrix metalloproteinase production by recombinant extracellular matrix metalloproteinase inducer from transfected Chinese hamster ovary cells. J Biol Chem. (1997). , 272, 24-27.

[244] Sameshima, T, Nabeshima, K, Toole, B. P, Yokogami, K, Okada, Y, Goya, T, Koono, M, & Wakisaka, S. Glioma cell extracellular matrix metalloproteinase inducer (EMMPRIN) (CD147)stimulates production of membrane-type matrix metalloproteinases and activated gelatinase A in co-cultures with brain-derived fibroblasts. Cancer Lett. (2000)., 157, 177-184.

[245] Hakomori, S. Tumor malignancy defined by aberrant glycosylation and sphingo(glyco)lipid metabolism. Cancer Res. (1996)., 56, 5309-5318.

[246] Sun, J, & Hemler, M. E. Regulation of MMP-1 and MMP-2 production through CD147/extracellular matrix metalloproteinase inducer interactions. Cancer Res. (2001)., 61, 2276-2281.

[247] Tang, W, Chang, S. B, & Hemler, M. E. Links between CD147 function, glycosylation, and caveolin-1. Mol Biol Cell. (2004)., 15, 4043-4050.

[248] Ochrietor, J. D, Moroz, T. P, Clamp, M. F, Timmers, A. M, Muramatsu, T, & Linser, P. J. Inactivation of the Basigin gene impairs normal retinal development and maturation. Vision Res. (2002)., 42, 447-453.

[249] Ochrietor, J. D, Moroz, T. P, Van Ekeris, L, Clamp, M. F, Jefferson, S. C, Decarvalho, A. C, Fadool, J. M, Wistow, G, Muramatsu, T, & Linser, P. J. Retina-specific expression of 5A11/Basigin-2, a member of the immunoglobulin gene superfamily. Invest Ophthalmol Vis Sci. (2003). , 44, 4086-4096.

[250] Hori, K, Katayama, N, Kachi, S, Kondo, M, Kadomatsu, K, Usukura, J, Muramatsu, T, Mori, S, & Miyake, Y. Retinal dysfunction in basigin deficiency. Invest Ophthalmol Vis Sci. (2000). , 41, 3128-3133.

[251] Ochrietor, J. D, Moroz, T. M, Kadomatsu, K, Muramatsu, T, & Linser, P. J. Retinal degeneration following failed photoreceptor maturation in 5A11/basigin null mice. Exp Eye Res. (2001). , 72, 467-477.

[252] Clamp, M. F, Ochrietor, J. D, Moroz, T. P, & Linser, P. J. Developmental analyses of 5A11/Basigin, 5A11/Basigin-2 and their putative binding partner MCT1 in the mouse eye. Exp Eye Res. (2004). , 78, 777-789.

[253] Taylor, P. M, Woodfield, R. J, Hodgkin, M. N, Pettitt, T. R, Martin, A, Kerr, D. J, & Wakelam, M. J. Breast cancer cell-derived EMMPRIN stimulates fibroblast MMP2 release through a phospholipase A(2) and 5-lipoxygenase catalyzed pathway. Oncogene. (2002). , 21, 5765-5772.

[254] Lim, M, Martinez, T, Jablons, D, Cameron, R, Guo, H, Toole, B, Li, J. D, & Basbaum, C. Tumor-derived EMMPRIN (extracellular matrix metalloproteinase inducer) stimulates collagenase transcription through MAPK FEBS Lett. (1998). , 38.

[255] Sidhu, S. S, Mengistab, A. T, & Tauscher, A. N. LaVail J, Basbaum C. The microvesicle as a vehicle for EMMPRIN in tumor-stromal interactions. Oncogene. (2004). , 23, 956-563.

[256] Seiki, M, Koshikawa, N, & Yana, I. Role of pericellular proteolysis by membrane-type 1 matrix metalloproteinase in cancer invasion and angiogenesis. Cancer Metastasis Rev. (2003). , 22, 129-143.

[257] ItohY; Seiki, M. MT1-MMP: a potent modifier of pericellular microenvironment. J Cell Physiol. (2006). , 206, 1-8.

[258] Egawa, N, Koshikawa, N, Tomari, T, Nabeshima, K, Isobe, T, & Seiki, M. Membrane type 1 matrix metalloproteinase (MT1-MMP/MMP-14) cleaves and releases a 22-kDa extracellular matrix metalloproteinase inducer (EMMPRIN) fragment from tumor cells. J Biol Chem. (2006). , 281, 37576-37585.

[259] Grossniklaus, H. E, Cingle, K. A, Yoon, I. D, Ketkar, N, Hernault, L, & Brown, N. S. Correlation of histologic dimensional reconstruction and confocal scanning laser microscopic imaging of choroidal neovascularization in eyes with age-related maculopathy. Archives of Ophthalmology. (2000). , 2.

[260] Killingsworth, M. C, Sarks, J. P, & Sarks, H. S. Macrophages related to Bruch's membrane in age-related macular degeneration. Eye. (1990). Pt 4):613-621.

[261] Miceli, M. V, Liles, M. R, & Newsome, D. A. Evaluation of oxidative processes in human pigment epithelial cells associated with retinal outer segment phagocytosis. Experimental Cell Research. (1994). , 214(1), 242-249.

[262] Tate Jr DJMiceli MV, Newsome DA. Phagocytosis and H2O2 induce catalase and metallothionein gene expression in human retinal pigment epithelial cells. Investigative Ophthalmology & Visual Science. (1995). , 36(7), 1271-1279.

[263] Tate, D. J, Miceli, M. V, & Newsome, D. A. Expression of metallothionein isoforms in human chorioretinal complex.Current Eye Research. (2002). , 24(1), 12-25.

[264] Parthasarathy, S, & Santanam, N. Mechanisms of oxidation, antioxidants, and atherosclerosis.Current Opinion in Lipidology (1994). , 5(5), 371-375.

[265] Katsuda, S, & Kaji, T. Atherosclerosis and extracellular matrix. Journal of atherosclerosis and thrombosis. (2003). , 10(5), 267-274.

[266] St-pierre, Y, Van Themsche, C, & Esteve, P. O. Emerging features in the regulation of MMP-9 gene expression for the development of novel molecular targets and therapeutic strategies. Current Drug Targets: Inflammation & Allergy. (2003). , 2(3), 206-215.

[267] Patel, M, & Chan, C. C. Immunopathological aspects of age-related macular degeneration. Semin Immunopathol. (2008).

[268] Haines, J. L, Hauser, M. A, Schmidt, S, Scott, W. K, Olson, L. M, Gallins, P, Spencer, K. L, Kwan, S. Y, Noureddine, M, Gilbert, J. R, Schnetz-boutaud, N, Agarwal, A, Postel, E. A, & Pericak-vance, M. A. Complement factor H variant increases the risk of age-related macular degeneration. Science. (2005). , 308, 419-421.

[269] Lommatzsch, A, Hermans, P, Muller, K. D, Bornfeld, N, & Bird, A. C. Pauleikhoff. Are low inflammatory reactions involved in exudative age-related macular degeneration? Morphological and immunhistochemical analysis of AMD associated with basal deposits. Graefes Arch Clin Exp Ophthalmol. (2008). , 246(6), 803-810.

[270] Hinton, D. R, He, S, & Lopez, P. F. Apoptosis in surgically excised choroidal neovascular membranes in age-related macular degeneration. Arch Ophthalmol. (1998). , 116(2), 203-209.

[271] Penfold, P. L, Killingsworth, M. C, & Sarks, S. H. Senile macular degeneration: the involvement of immunocompetent cells. Graefes Arch Clin Exp Ophthalmol. (1985). , 223(2), 69-76.

[272] Penfold, P, Killingsworth, M, & Sarks, S. An ultrastructural study of the role of leucocytes and fibroblasts in the breakdown of Bruch's membrane. Aust J Ophthalmol. (1984). , 12(1), 23-31.

[273] Lopez, P. F, Grossniklaus, H. E, Lambert, H. M, Aaberg, T. M, & Capone, A. Sternberg P Jr, L'Hernault N. Pathologic features of surgically excised subretinal neovas-

cular membranes in age-related macular degeneration. Am J Ophthalmol. (1991). , 112(6), 647-656.

[274] Ibrahim, M, Chair, B, & Kartz, D. The injured cells: the role of dendritic cell system as a sentinel receptor pathway. Immunol Today. (1995). , 16, 181-186.

[275] Matyszak, M, & Perry, V. The potential role of dendritic cells in immune-mediated inflammatory diseases in the central nervous system. Neuroscience. (1996). , 74, 599-608.

[276] Luft, F. C, Mervaala, E, Muller, D. N, Gross, V, Schmidt, F, Joon, K. P, et al. Hypertension-induced end-organ damage: a new transgenic approach to an old problem. Hypertension. (1999). , 33, 212-218.

[277] Alexander, R. W. Hypertension and the pathogenesis of atherosclerosis: oxidative stress and the mediation of arterial inflammatory response, a new perspective. Hypertension. (1995). , 25, 155-161.

[278] Yla-herttuala, S, Lipton, B. A, Rosenfeld, M. E, Srakioja, T, Yoshimura, T, & Leonard, E. J. Expression of monocyte chemoattractant protein-1 in macrophage-rich areas of human and rabbit atherosclerotic lesions. Proc Natl Acad Sci USA.(1991). , 88, 5252-5256.

[279] Yu X Dluz SGraves DT, Zhang L, Antoniades HN, Hollander W. Elevated expression of monocyte chemoattractant protein-1 by vascular smooth muscle cells in hypercholesterolemic primates. Proc Natl Acad Sci USA. (1992). , 89, 6953-6957.

[280] Capers, Q, Alexander, R. W, Lou, P, De Leon, H, Wilcox, J. N, & Ishizaka, N. Monocyte chemoattractant protein-1 expression in aortic tissues of hypertensive rats. Hypertension. (1997). , 30, 1397-1402.

[281] BehrTM; Wang, XK; Aijar, N; Coatney, RW; Li, X; Koster, P. Monocyte chemoattractant protein-1 is upregulated in rats with volume overloaded congestive heart failure. Circulation, (2000). , 102, 1315-1322.

[282] Hilgers, K. F, Hartner, A, Porst, M, Mai, M, Wittmann, M, & Hugo, C. Monocyte chemoattractant protein-1 and macrophage infiltration in hypertensive kidney injury. Kidney Int. (2000). , 58, 2408-2419.

[283] Hernandez-presa, M, Bustos, C, Ortego, M, Tunon, J, Renedo, G, Ruiz-ortega, M, & Egido, J. Angiotensin-converting enzyme inhibition prevents arterial nuclear factor-kappa B activation, monocyte chemoattractant protein-1 expression, and macrophage infiltration in a rabbit model of early accelerated atherosclerosis. Circulation. (1997). , 95, 1532-1541.

[284] Ruiz-ortega, M, Ruperez, M, Lorenzo, O, Esteban, V, Blanco, J, & Mezzano, S. Angiotensin II regulates the synthesis of proinflammatory cytokines and chemokines in the kidney. Kidney Int. (2002). suppl 82):12-22.

[285] Tham, D. M. Martin-McNulty B, Wang YX, Wilson DW, Vergona R, Sullivan ME. Angiotensin II is associated with activation of NF-kappa B-mediated genes and downregulation of PPARs. Physiol Genom. (2002). , 11, 21-31.

[286] Yoshimura, T, & Leonard, E. J. Identification of high affinity receptors for human monocyte chemoattractant protein-1 on human monocytes. J Immunol. (1990). , 145, 292-297.

[287] Charo, I. F, Myers, S. J, Herman, A, Franci, C, Connolly, A. J, & Coughlin, S. R. Molecular cloning and functional expression of two monocyte chemoattractant protein-1 receptors reveals alternative splicing of the carboxyl-terminal trails. Proc Natl Acad Sci USA. (1994). , 91, 2752-2756.

[288] Uetama, T, Ohno-matsui, K, Nakahama, K, Morita, I, & Mochizuki, M. Phenotypic change regulates monocyte chemoattractant protein-1 (MCP-1) gene expression in human retinal pigment epithelial cells. J Cell Physiol. (2003). , 197, 77-85.

[289] Higgins, G. T, Wang, J. H, Dockery, P, Cleary, P. E, & Redmond, H. P. Induction of angiogenic cytokine expression in cultured RPE by ingestion of oxidized photoreceptor outer segments. Invest Ophthalmol Vis Sci. (2003). , 44, 1775-1782.

[290] Ambati, J, Anand, A, Fernandez, S, Sakurai, E, Lynn, B. C, Kuziel, W. A, Rollins, B. J, & Ambati, B. K. An animal model of age-related macular degeneration in senescent Ccl-2- or Ccr-2-deficient mice. Nat Med. (2003). , 9, 1390-1397.

[291] Tuo, J, Bojanowski, C. M, Zhou, M, Shen, D, Ross, R. J, Rosenberg, K. I, Cameron, D. J, Yin, C, Kowalak, J. A, Zhuang, Z, Zhang, K, & Chan, C. C. Murine ccl2/cx3cr1 deficiency results in retinal lesions mimicking human age-related macular degeneration. Invest Ophthalmol Vis Sci. (2007). , 48, 3827-3836.

[292] Holtkamp, G. M, De Vos, A. F, Peek, R, & Kijlsta, A. Analysis of the secretion pattern of monocyte chemotactic protein-1 (MCP-1) and transforming growth factor-beta 2 (TGF-beta2) by human retinal pigment epithelial cells. Clin Exp Immunol. (1999). , 118, 35-40.

[293] Zheng, J, Singh, S, Fan, W, & Mclaughlin, B. Gene expression in human retinal pigment epithelial cells (ARPE-19) during wound healing. Exp Eye Res (Suppl). (2000). S113.

[294] Pons, M, & Marin-castano, M. E. Cigarette smoke-related hydroquinone dysregulates MCP-1, VEGF and PEDF expression in retinal pigment epithelium in vitro and in vivo. PLoS ONE, (2011). e16722.

[295] Behr, T. M, Willette, R. N, Coatney, R. W, Berova, M, Angermann, C. E, & Anderson, K. Eprosartan improves cardiac performance, reduces cardiac hypertrophy and mortality and downregulates myocardial MCP-1 and inflammation in hypertensive heart disease. J Hypertens. (2004). , 22, 583-592.

[296] Basso, N, Paglia, N, Stella, I, De Cavanagh, E. M, Ferder, L, Arnaiz, M, & Inserra, F. Protective effect of the inhibition of the renin-angiotensis system on aging. Regul Pept. (2005). , 128, 247-252.

[297] Diz, D, & Lewis, K. Dahl memorial lecture: the renin-angiotensisn system and aging. Hypertension. (2008). , 52, 37-43.

[298] Funakoshi, Y, Ichiki, T, Shimokawa, H, Egashira, K, Takeda, K, & Kaibuchi, K. Rho-kinase mediates angiotensin II-induced monocyte chemoattractant protein-1 expression in rat vascular smooth muscle cells. Hypertension, (2001). , 38, 100-104.

[299] Wu, L, Iwai, M, Nakagami, H, Li, Z, Chen, R, & Suzuki, J. Roles of angiotensin II type 2 receptor stimulation associated with selective angiotensin II type 1 receptor blockade with valsartan in the improvement of inflammation-induced vascular injury. Circulation, (2001). , 104, 2716-2721.

[300] Sozzani, S, Luini, W, Molino, M, Jilek, P, Bottazzi, B, & Cerletti, C. The signaling transduction pathway involved in the migration induced by a monocyte chemotactic cytokine. J Immunol. (1991). , 147, 2215-2221.

[301] Chen, X. L, Tummala, P. E, Olbrych, M. T, Alexander, R. W, & Medford, R. M. Angiotensin II induces monocyte chemoattractant protein-1 gene expression in rat vascular smooth muscle cells. Circ Res. (1998). , 83, 952-959.

[302] Locati, M, Zhou, D, Luini, W, Evangelista, V, Mantovani, A, & Sozzani, S. Rapid induction of arachidonic acid release by monocyte chemotactic protein-1 and related chemokines: role of Ca^{2+} influx, synergism with platelet-activating factor and significance for chemotaxis. J Biol Chem. (1994). , 269, 4746-4753.

[303] Yu, B. P, & Chung, H. Y. Adaptive mechanisms to oxidative stress during aging. Mech Ageing Dev. (2006). , 127, 436-443.

[304] Kim, H. J, Jung, K. J, Yu, B. P, Cho, C. G, Choi, J. S, & Chung, H. Y. Modulation of redox-sensitive transcription factors by calorie restriction during aging. Mech Ageing Dev. (2002). , 123, 1589-1595.

[305] Chung, H. Y, Kim, H. J, Kim, K. W, Choi, J. S, & Yu, B. P. Molecular inflammation hypothesis of aging based on the anti-aging mechanism of calorie restriction. Microsc Res Tech. (2002). , 59, 264-272.

[306] Miyata, N, Yamakoshi, Y, & Nakanishi, I. Reactive species responsible for biological actions of photo excited fullerenes. Yakugaku Zasshi. (2002). , 120, 1007-1016.

[307] Murkies, A. Phytoestrogens what is the current knowledge? Aust Fam Physician. (1998). SS51, 47.

[308] Joly, S, Samardzija, M, Wenzel, A, Thiersch, M, & Grimm, C. Nonessential role of beta3 and beta5 integrin subunits for efficient clearance of cellular debris after light-induced photoreceptor degeneration. Invest Ophthalmol Vis Sci. (2009). , 50, 423-1432.

[309] Ohno-matsui, K, Morita, I, Tombran-tink, J, Mrazek, D, & Onodera, M. Novel mechanism for age-related macular degeneration: an equilibrium shift between the angiogenesis factors VEGF and PEDF. J Cell Physiol. (2001). , 189, 323-333.

[310] Adamis, A. P, Shima, D. T, Yeo, K. T, Yeo, T. K, Brown, L. F, Berse, B, Amore, D, Folkman, P. A, & Synthesis, J. and secretion of vascular permeability factor/vascular endothelial growth factor by human retinal pigment epithelial cells. Biochem Biophys Res Commun. (1993). , 193, 631-638.

[311] Husain, D, Ambati, B, Adamis, A. P, & Miller, J. W. Mechanisms of age-related macular degeneration. Ophthalmol Clin North Am. (2002). , 15, 87-91.

[312] Kwak, N, Okamoto, N, Wood, J. M, & Campochiaro, P. A. VEGF is major stimulator in model of choroidal neovascularization. Invest Ophthalmol Vis Sci. (2000). , 41, 3158-3164.

[313] Tong, J. P, & Yao, Y. F. Contribution of VEGF and PEDF to choroidal angiogenesis: a need for balanced expressions. Clin Biochem. (2006). , 39, 267-276.

[314] Witmer, A. N, Vrensen, G. F, Van Noorden, C. J, & Schlingemann, R. O. Vascular endothelial growth actors and angiogenesis in eye disease. Prog Retin Eye Res. (2003). , 22, 1-29.

[315] Kliffen, M, Sharma, H. S, Mooy, C. M, Kerkvliet, S, & De Jong, P. T. Increased expression of angiogenic growth factors in age-related maculopathy. Br J Ophthalmol. (1997). , 81, 54-162.

[316] Kvanta, A, Algvere, P. V, Berglin, L, & Seregard, S. Subfoveal fibrovascular membranes in age-related macular degeneration express vascular endothelial growth factor. Invest Ophthalmol Vis Sci. (1996). , 37, 1929-1934.

[317] Lopez, P. F, Sippy, B. D, Lambert, H. M, Thach, A. B, & Hinton, D. R. Transdifferentiated retinal pigment epithelial cells are immunoreactive for vascular endothelial growth factor in surgically excised age-related macular degeneration-related choroidal neovascular membranes. Invest Ophthalmol Vis Sci. (1996). , 37, 855-868.

[318] Reich, S. J, Fosnot, J, Kuroki, A, Tang, W, Yang, X, Maguire, A. M, Bennett, J, & Tolentino, M. J. Small interfering RNA (siRNA) targeting VEGF effectively inhibits ocular neovascularization in a mouse model. Mol Vis. (2003). , 9-210.

[319] Olsson, A. K, Dimberg, A, Kreuger, J, & Claesson-welsh, L. VEGF receptor signalling- in control of vascular function. Nat Rev Mol Cell Biol. (2006). , 7, 59-371.

[320] Yi, X, Ogata, N, Komada, M, Yamamoto, C, Takahashi, K, Omori, K, & Uyama, M. Vascular endothelial growth factor expression in choroidal neovascularization in rats. Graefes Arch Clin Exp Ophthalmol. (1997). , 235, 313-319.

[321] Dawson, D. W, Volpert, O. V, Gillis, P, Crawford, S. E, Xu, H, Benedict, W, & Bouck, N. P. Pigment epithelium-derived factor: a potent inhibitor of angiogenesis. Science, (1999). , 285, 245-248.

[322] Bhutto, I. A, Mcleod, D. S, Hasegawa, T, Kim, S. Y, Merges, C, Tong, P, & Lutty, G. A. Pigment epithelium-derived factor (PEDF) and vascular endothelial growth factor (VEGF) in aged human choroid and eyes with age-related macular degeneration. Exp Eye Res. (2006). , 82, 99-110.

[323] Ogata, N, Wada, M, Otsuji, T, Jo, N, Tombran-tink, J, & Matsumura, M. Expression of pigment epithelium-derived factor in normal adult rat eye and experimental choroidal neovascularization. Invest Ophthalmol Vis Sci. (2002). , 43, 1168-1175.

[324] Holekamp, N. M, Bouck, N, & Volpert, O. Pigment epithelium-derived factor is deficient in the vitreous of patients with choroidal neovascularization due to age-related macular degeneration. Am J Ophthalmol. (2002). , 134, 220-227.

[325] Bamias, G, & Martin, C. rd, Marini M, et al: Expression, localization, and functional activity of TL1A, a novel Th1-polarizing cytokine in inflammatory bowel disease. J Immunol (2003). , 171, 4868-4874.

[326] Prehn, J. L, Mehdizadeh, S, Landers, C. J, et al. Potential role for TL1A, the new TNF-family member and potent costimulator of IFN-gamma, in mucosal inflammation. Clin Immunol (2004). , 112, 66-77.

[327] Al-lamki, R. S, Wang, J, Tolkovsky, A. M, et al. TL1A both promotes and protects from renal inflammation and injury. J Am Soc Nephrol (2008). , 19, 953-960.

[328] Bamias, G, Siakavellas, S. I, Stamatelopoulos, K. S, Chryssochoou, E, & Papamichael, C. and Sfikakis PP: Circulating levels of TNF-like cytokine 1A (TL1A) and its decoy receptor 3 (DcR3) in rheumatoid arthritis. Clin Immunol. (2008). , 129, 249-255.

[329] Zhang, N, Sanders, A. J, Ye, L, & Jiang, W. G. Vascular endothelial growth inhibitor in human cancer (Review). Int J of Molecular Medicone. (2008). , 24, 3-8.

[330] Deng, W, Gu, X, Lu, Y, Gu, C, Zheng, Y, Zhang, Z, Chen, L, Yao, Z, & Li, L. Y. Down-modulation of TNFSF15 in ovarian cancer by VEGF and MCP-1 is a pre-requisite for tumor neovascularization. Angiogenesis. (2011). Dec 31. (Epub ahead of print

[331] Apte, R. S, Barreiro, R. A, Duh, E, Volpert, O, & Ferguson, T. A. Stimulation of neovascularization by the anti-angiogenic factor PEDF. Invest Ophthalmol Vis Sci. (2004). , 45, 4491-4497.

[332] Ohno-matsui, K, Yoshida, T, Uetama, T, Mochizuki, M, & Morita, I. Vascular endothelial growth factor upregulates pigment epithelium-derived factor expression via VEGFR-1 in human retinal pigment epithelial cells. Biochem Biophys Res Commun. (2003). , 303, 962-967.

[333] Pons, M, & Marin-castaño, M. E. Nicotine increases the VEGF/PEDF ratio in retinal pigment epithelium: a possible mechanism for CNV in passive smokers with AMD. Invest Ophthalmol Vis Sci. (2011). , 52(6), 3842-53.

[334] Fang, L, Chen, M. F, Xiao, Z. L, Yu, G. L, Chen, X. B, & Xie, X. M. The Effect of Endothelial Progenitor Cells on Angiotensin II-induced Proliferation of Cultured Rat Vascular Smooth Muscle Cells. J Cardiovasc Pharmacol. (2011). , 58(6), 617-25.

[335] Guo, R. W, Yang, L. X, Li, M. Q, Pan, X. H, Liu, B, & Deng, Y. L. Stimand Orai1-mediated store-operated calcium entry is critical for angiotensin II-induced vascular smooth muscle cell proliferation. Cardiovasc Res. (2012). Jan 2. (Epub ahead of print), 1.

[336] Yang, L. L, Li, D. Y, Zhang, Y. B, Zhu, M. Y, Chen, D, & Xu, T. D. Salvianolic acid A inhibits angiotensin II-induced proliferation of human umbilical vein endothelial cells by attenuating the production of ROS. Acta Pharmacol Sin. 2012 Jan; doi:aps. (2011). Epub 2011 Nov 21., 33(1), 41-8.

[337] Zhu, N, Zhang, D, Chen, S, Liu, X, Lin, L, Huang, X, Guo, Z, Liu, J, Wang, Y, Yuan, W, & Qin, Y. Endothelial enriched microRNAs regulate angiotensin II-induced endothelial inflammation and migration. Atherosclerosis. (2011). , 215(2), 286-93.

[338] Martini, A, Bruno, R, Mazzulla, S, Nocita, A, & Martino, G. Angiotensin II regulates endothelial cell migration through calcium influx via T-type calcium channel in human umbilical vein endothelial cells. Acta Physiol (Oxf). (2010). , 198(4), 449-55.

[339] Montiel, M, De La Blanca, E. P, & Jiménez, E. Angiotensin II induces focal adhesion kinase/paxillin phosphorylation and cell migration in human umbilical vein endothelial cells. Biochem Biophys Res Commun. (2005). , 327(4), 971-8.

[340] Nadal, J. A, Scicli, G. M, Carbini, L. A, & Scicli, A. G. Angiotensin II stimulates migration of retinal microvascular pericytes: involvement of TGF-beta and PDGF-BB. Am J Physiol Heart Circ Physiol. (2002). H , 739-48.

[341] Buharalioglu, C. K, Song, C. Y, Yaghini, F. A, Ghafoor, H. U, Motiwala, M, Adris, T, Estes, A. M, & Malik, K. U. Angiotensin II-induced process of angiogenesis is mediated by spleen tyrosine kinase via VEGF receptor-1 phosphorylation. Am J Physiol Heart Circ Physiol. (2011). H , 1043-55.

[342] Benndorf, R, Böger, R. H, Ergün, S, Steenpass, A, & Wieland, T. Angiotensin II type 2 receptor inhibits vascular endothelial growth factor-induced migration and in vitro tube formation of human endothelial cells. Circ Res. (2003). , 93(5), 438-47.

[343] Espinosa-HeidmannDG; Sall, J; Hernandez, EP; Cousins, SW. Basal laminar deposit formation in APO B100 transgenic mice: complex interactions between dietary fat, blue light, and vitamin E. Invest Ophthalmol Vis Sci. (2004). , 45(1), 260-266.

[344] Pons, M, Cousins, S. W, Alcazar, O, Striker, G. E, & Marin-castaño, M. E. Angiotensin II-induced MMP-2 activity and MMP-14 and basigin protein expression are mediated via the angiotensin II receptor type 1-mitogen-activated protein kinase 1 pathway in retinal pigment epithelium implications for age-related macular degeneration. Am J Pathol. (2011). , 178(6), 2665-81.

Section 2

Classification, Clinical Features and New Advance in OCT Diagnosis

Chapter 3

Classification and Clinical Features of AMD

Petr Kolar

Additional information is available at the end of the chapter

http://dx.doi.org/10.5772/53762

1. Introduction

Disease was first time described as "Symmetrical central choroido-retinal disease occurring in senile persons" in 1874 by Hutchinson. About 25 years ago, the term "age-related maculopathy" was accepted and end stage of disease was acknowledged as age-related macular degeneration [1]. AMD is leading cause of blindness worldwide in older patient population. The highest risk of developing of AMD is in the population older than 65 years. With ageing of population in many countries, more than 20 % might have the disease [2]. Advanced forms of AMD are associated with visual progressive impairment. Visual acuity of this subjects decreases to practical blindness. This has big socioeconomic impact.

AMD is progressive chronic disease that is located in central retinal area (macula luthea – yellow spot) [2]. Most visual lost is identified in late stages of AMD. There are 2 categories: wet AMD and geographic atrophy. In wet AMD choroidal neovascularization breaks through neuroretina. Leaking vessels, hemorrhages and lipid deposits lead to scarring process in macular area. All retinal structures including photoreceptors are destroyed. In geographic atrophy occur progressive atrophy of retinal pigment epithelium and secondary photoreceptors. To the end of 20th century was AMD practically untreatable. However, new pharmaceuticals based on suppression of vascular endothelial growth factor (VEGF) have completely changed the treatment of the disease [2]. Nearly 95 % of patients can be prevented from visual lost, and nearly 40 % of them improve vision [2].

2. Epidemiology, risk factors, and natural history

Prevalence and incidence

In last 30 years were published many epidemiological studies on AMD. In a meta-analysis of population-based studies in white people aged 40 years and older, the prevalence of early age-related macular degeneration was estimated to be 6.8% and late age-related macular degeneration 1.5%[3].

Results from the Baltimore Eye Study reported epidemiological data from other ethnic groups. Late AMD was nine to ten times more prevalent in white participants than in black ones [4]. Age-specific prevalence of late age-related macular degeneration in Asians is largely similar to that in white people [5].

In Asia population have often disease specific features. Many of them have polypoidal dilatation of the choroidal vasculature. Polypoidal choroidal vasculopathy can account for 50% of wet AMD cases in Asians, but only 8-13% in white people [5].

Another variant of AMD is retinal angiomatous proliferation (RAP), which accounts for 12-15% of neovascular age-related macular degeneration [6]. RAP usually not responds to standard management of wet AMD.

There are few incidence studies on AMD. The US Beaver Dam Eye Study in the USA reported a 14.3% 15-year cumulative incidence for early AMD and 3.1% for late AMD in adults aged 43-86 years [7].

3. Risk factors of AMD

The major risk factor for AMD is older age. More than 10% of people older than 80 years have late AMD. Female sex has been inconsistently reported as a risk factor as well [3].

The major systemic risk factors include cigarette smoking [8]. Cigarette smoking in particular is a strong and consistent risk factor for AMD. Smoking 20 cigarettes a day increases the risk of double. Obesity is further systemic risk factor. This is connected with systemic riscs of obesity. These patients are more likely to have hypertension and diabetes mellitus, which are another risk factors [9,10]. People with AMD are also at increased risk of stroke [11].

Ocular risk factors for age-related macular degeneration include darker iris pigmentation, previous cataract surgery, and hyperopic refraction. A meta-analysis suggested previous cataract surgery was a strong risk factor for age-related macular degeneration, but this association was not shown in a randomized clinical trial [12].

Table 1 summarizes the risk factors for age-related macular degeneration.

4. Genetic factors

Last ten years several genes have been associated to have role in pathogenesis of AMD [2].

AMD is disease that is tightly connected with inflammatory reaction. Inflammatory and immunologic processes play major role in its pathogenesis. For this reason was identified complement factor H gene (CFH). Other confirmed genes in the complement pathway include

http://dx.doi.org/10.5772/53762

C2, CFB, C3 and CFI.29-31. On the basis of large genome-wide association studies, HDL cholesterol pathway genes have been implicated, including LIPC and CETP, and possibly ABCA1 and LPL.32-34 APOE in the LDL pathway might also be related to AMD [13]. The collagen matrix pathway genes COL10A1 and COL8A1 and the extracellular matrix pathway gene TIMP3 have also been linked to age-related macular degeneration [14]. Finally, genes in the angiogenesis pathway (VEGFA) have also been associated with age-related macular degeneration in a meta-analysis of two AMD genome-wide association studies [14].

Older age, female sex
Cigarette smoking
Obesity, Hypertension, Diabetes mellitus
Low dietary intake of vitamins A, C, and E, and zinc
Low dietary intake of lutein and omega-3 fatty acids
Unhealthy lifestyle related to cardiovascular risk factors

Table 1. Risk factors for age-related macular degeneration (adapted from [2])

Genes modifying several biological pathways are in AMD. Complement and immune processes, HDL cholesterol, and mechanisms involving collagen, extra-cellular matrix, and angiogenesis pathways are associated with the onset, progression, and bilateral involvement of AMD [2]. But it should be noted that genetic susceptibility can be modified by environmental factors. Genetic variations can also influence differential responses to treatments for age-related macular degeneration, an emerging research area [2].

Table 2 summarizes major genes associated with onset and progression of AMD

5. Clinical manifestations of the process of natural retinal aging

Aging is a physiological process involving all body organs and tissues. This process also affects the eye. It is a physiological process. That is not a manifestation of any disease. Each body cell has a planned life cycle from its inception to apoptosis (cell death). Body tissue in which there is no restoration of extinct mitotic cells (nerve tissue, retina), have a high incidence of manifestations of aging especially after the 75th year of life.

Clinical manifestation of retinal aging is mainly visible as a foveal reflex loss. Its background is in the loss of cells from the inner retinal layers around the foveola and extending of foveal avascular zone [15]. In macular zone are usually present small hard drusen, which are not yet a manifestation of AMD [16]. In macula also occur tigers like irregularities in pigmentation. Visual acuity remains on a physiological level unlike of subjects affected by AMD. Doppler velocimetry demonstrates decrease of blood flow to the macular area [17]. Further is detectable reduction of perifoveolar arterioles and venules together with enlargement of foveal avascular zone [18] and reduction of retinal ganglion cells amount [19].

Also can be diagnosed decrease of other visual functions in connection with the process of aging. There are especially adaptation to darkness, contrast sensitivity, color vision and ability of stereopsis [20].

CFH (complement factor H; chr 1)
ABCA4 (ATP-binding cassette transporter; chr 1)
COL8A1 (collagen type 8 alpha 1 subunit; chr 3)
CF1 (complement factor 1; chr 4)
VEGFA (vascular endothelial growth factor A; chr 6)
FRK/COL10A1 (fyn-related kinase/alpha chain of type X collagen; chr 6)
CFB (complement factor B [properdin]; chr 6)
C2 (complement component 2; chr 6)
ARMS2/HTRA1 (HtrA-serinepeptidase1; chr 10)
LIPC (hepatic lipase; chr 15)
CETP (cholesterylester transfer protein; chr 16)
APOE (apolipoprotein E; chr 19)
C3 (complement component 3; chr 19)
TIMP3 (tissue inhibitor of metalloproteinase 3; chr 22)
TNFRSF10A (tumor necrosis factor receptor superfamily 10a; chr 8)

Table 2. Summery of genes studied according to their impact on AMD (adapted from [2])

6. Classification and clinical features of age-related macular degeneration

Age-related macular degeneration can be divided into 2 categories: dry form (non-exudative) and wet form (exudative). The dry form is very prevalent and affects about 85 to 90 % of patients. The wet form occurs in the remaining 10 to 15 %. Impairment of central visual acuity is much higher in wet form of AMD than in dry form. Wet form is responsible for 85 % of severe vision loss.

6.1. Dry form of AMD

The dry form of AMD occurs independently on the choroidal neovascular membrane (CNV). It is associated with chorioretinal atrophy with no obvious defects in Bruch's membrane. Clinical studies show a decrease in chorioretinal blood flow [21]. Chorioretinal atrophy leads to subsequent degeneration of the retinal pigment epithelium cells (RPE). It is associated with involution of photoreceptors in the affected area [22]. The dry form of AMD includes atrophy of the outer part of hematoretinal barrier (HRB) without appreciable leakage. It seems that the barrier function is maintained and the area of atrophy remains dry.

Both forms of AMD are presented with painless loss of central vision. Individuals with dry AMD will typically complain of blurred vision as well as difficulty seeing fine details clearly. In the advanced stages, atrophic macular areas often coalesce, creating central scotoma, or blind spots, in the central visual field. This central visual loss compromises an individual's ability to perform basic tasks such as recognizing faces, reading signs, and other activities of daily living. Individuals with wet AMD will commonly present with visual distortion in which straight lines appear deformed. A hallmark of conversion from dry to wet AMD is a sudden and profound loss or distortion of central vision. These visual changes occur as a result of the acute degenerative changes occurring in the macula - most notably, subretinal and intraretinal hemorrhages from choroidal neovascular membrane. Individuals will typically have preserved peripheral vision in both processes [23].

6.2. Dry AMD

Dry AMD, the more common variety of the AMD, results from degeneration of outer retinal cells (RPE cells) with subsequent profound retinal dysfunction (damage of photoreceptors and retinal neurons).

The dry form of the disease is usually asymptomatic. Progression to the wet form may be indicated by sudden, severe vision loss or new onset of visual distortion (metamorphopsia).

The dry form of the disease is characterized by macular drusen, however alterations in RPE are visible. Intermediate to severe cases of the dry form are characterized by larger drusen and geographic atrophy of RPE layer. This can cause severe vision loss [24].

Regular examinations are important to determine whether patients may benefit from certain interventions. For patients over age 55 with no risk factors, a comprehensive eye exam every one to two years is recommended. Patients with early-stage disease or a family history of the condition may require closer follow-up. Those with an intermediate or advanced case of the dry form of the disease should be advised to take a particular combination multivitamin recommended in the Age-Related Eye Disease Study. These supplements reduce the risk of progression to the wet form of the disease by 25%. However, patients with early-stage disease may not benefit from such supplementation. Smoking cessation is associated with a substantial reduction in the risk of progression to late-stage disease [24].

Self-monitoring with an Amsler grid (available online at www.macula.org/amsler-grid) is critical and can help detect disease progression as early as possible. New onset of visual distortion noted on an Amsler grid, or any other sudden change in vision, may indicate progression from dry to the wet form of AMD. In some cases, timely treatment can reduce the risk of permanent loss of vision [24].

Patients who describe a sudden change in vision should be referred for urgent ophthalmic evaluation [24].

Drusen

In early dry AMD, various lipid and protein-rich extracellular deposits accumulate under the RPE [25]. Clinically, deposits of AMD are classified on fundoscopic features of morphology and size.

Drusen are a marker of age-related macular degeneration (AMD). Lesions similar to drusen, both in histology and their clinical appearance, are also seen in choroidal tumours, chronic inflammatory and degenerative conditions of the eye. Drusen are yellowish-white deposits of extracellular material located between the retinal pigment epithelium (RPE) and the inner collagenous zone of Bruch's membrane. They are the result of ageing. Drusen seen in these varied conditions have a similar clinical and histological appearance [26].

As seen through the ophthalmoscope, drusen are dots ranging in color from white to yellow, sometimes with a crystalline, glittering aspect. The origin of drusen has remained unresolved for more than a century. Moreover, there is no agreement as to whether drusen in the absence of other ocular abnormalities always point to early age-related macular degeneration [1].

Inside Bruch's membrane we can differentiate several biochemical and anatomical changes with aging, including collagenous thickening, calcification, and lipid infiltration, in the absence of apparent retinal dysfunction. The accumulation of specific deposits under the RPE is the hallmark histopathological feature of eyes with early AMD, when visual function is still not irreversibly impaired. Histopathological examination defines three main types of sub-RPE deposits on the basis of location, thickness, and content: basal laminar deposits (BLamD), basal linear deposits (BLinD), and nodular drusen. BLamD is seen as amorphous material of intermediate electron density between the plasma membrane and the basement membrane of the RPE, often containing banded structures (wide-spaced collagen), patches of electron-dense fibrillar or granular material, and occasionally, membranous debris [27]. They are distributed throughout the retina, including the periphery as well as the macula, underlying not only cones but rods as well. BLinD are diffuse, amorphous accumulations within the inner collagenous zone of BrM, external to RPE basement membrane, with similar content variations [Green]. BLinD are characterized by coated and non-coated vesicles as well as some membranous and empty profiles [28]. Biochemically, deposits contain phospholipids, triglycerides, cholesterol, cholesterol esters, unsaturated fatty acids, peroxidized lipids, and apolipoproteins [29].

In contrast to BLamD and BLinD, nodular drusen are discrete, dome-shaped deposits within the inner collagenous zone of BrM (i.e., external to the RPE basal lamina). Due to their location, nodular drusen are often contiguous with BLinD, and can be difficult to distinguish

http://dx.doi.org/10.5772/53762

from BLinD without electron microscopy [25]. Differences between BLamD and BLinD are seen on Figure 1.

A key factor influencing the classification of drusen is their size and shape. Simple aids, the widest diameter of venous branches at the edge of the disc, which has a dimension of 125 microns, determine the size of drusen.

Drusen are classified according to their appearance and size in the two basic categories:

1. Hard drusen

Their size is smaller than 63 microns. Ophthalmoscopic examination shows us small and well-demarcated yellow deposits (Figure 2.). This type of drusen is associated with very low risk of progression to late forms of AMD. However the occurrence of more than 8 hard drusen is associated with an increased risk of occurrence soft drusen.

2. Soft drusen: their size is greater than 63 microns are not sharply defined; often coalesce (Figure 3.). They are associated with higher risk of developing of wet AMD. If they affect foveal region they are often associated with the occurrence of metamorphopsia on Amsler grid. Over time, soft drusen can confluent and form irregular detachment of the RPE.

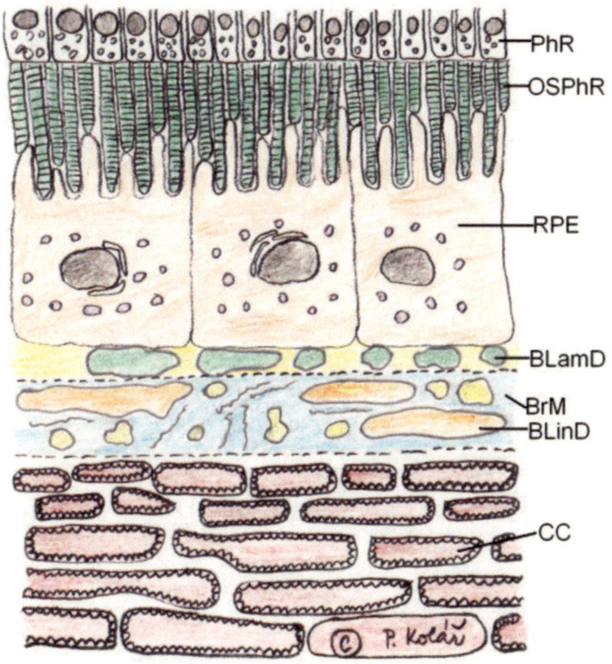

Figure 1. Schema of drusen in AMD. Legend: PhR – Photoreceptor, OSPhR – Outer Segment of Photoreceptor, RPE – Retinal Pigment Epithelium, BLamD – Basal Laminar Deposits, BLinD – Basal Linear Deposits, BrM – Bruch's Membrane, CC – Choriocapillaris

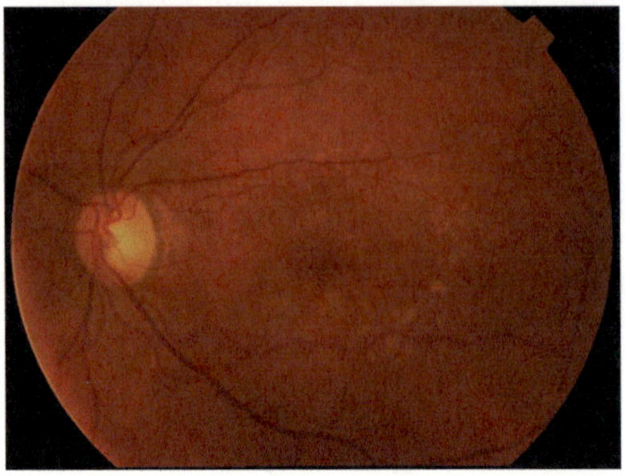

Figure 2. Hard drusen in macular region

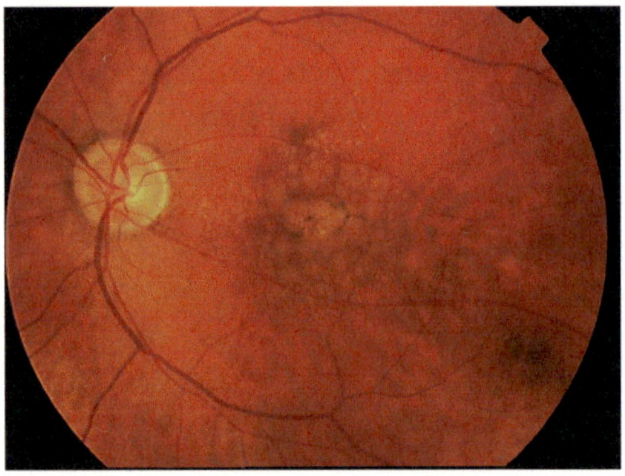

Figure 3. Soft drusen in macular region

Occurrence of drusen, however, is not a static phenomenon. Their presence is characterized by dynamic changes. Hard drusen can grow and change to soft drusen. Soft drusen can grow and coalesce into large confluent bodies. This leads to detachment of the RPE. Another change that can be seen is calcification. Inside drusen are visible cholesterol crystals. Drusen with advancing age usually increased in their amount. Presence of soft drusen in both eyes is an important risk factor in the development of advanced forms of AMD (geographic atrophy of the RPE and CNV). Hard drusen are, however, frequently associated with the occurrence of dry AMD [30].

Changes in retinal pigment epithelium

Irregularities in the RPE are associated with all stages of AMD. Focal hyperpigmentation arises from changes at the level of the RPE. We can differentiate hyperpigmentation or RPE cells, proliferation or migration of RPE cells into the subretinal space (Figure 4.). Focal hyperpigmentation is commonly associated with chorioretinal anastomosis.

http://dx.doi.org/10.5772/53762

Focal hypopigmentation is associated with areas of drusen, which leads to thinning of the RPE cells layer and reduction of melanin content. Low melanin content is associated with a high risk of transition to the wet form of AMD.

Geographic atrophy of RPE cells

Geographic atrophy (GA) of RPE is end-stage dry AMD. GA is characterized by well-circumscribed area of RPE atrophy, which allows good visualization of the choroid and in end stage of disease sclera (Figure 5., Figure 6.). The term geographic atrophy is not accurate name for this stage, because it is not only RPE atrophy, but also choriocapilaris and retinal atrophy. These three layers are inseparably joined together. The atrophy of one of them leads to irreversible atrophy of the other twos. GA can occurs either as a primary form of AMD, or followed by a secondary form after absorption of soft drusen, after flattening of RPE detachment, or as a consequence of CNV regression, or rupture of the RPE. GA of RPE is causing severe loss of visual acuity in 20% of AMD patients. The remaining 80% of the severe losses of visual acuity in AMD is caused by CNV.

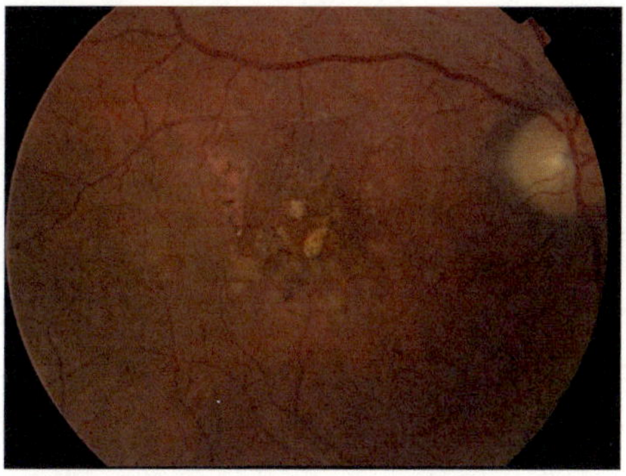

Figure 4. Hyperpigmentation and proliferation of RPE cells

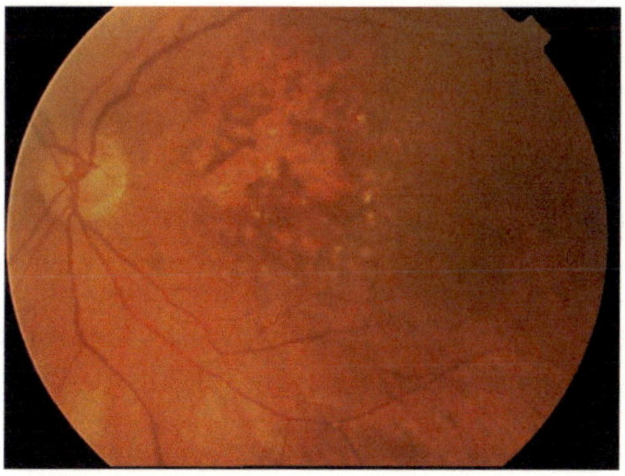

Figure 5. Geographic atrophy of RPE (color image)

Patients with primary GA are on average older than patients with wet AMD. Based on these circumstances, it has been suggested that the GA process occurs as reaction to changes in Bruch's membrane in those eyes, which are not developed wet form of AMD.

Patients with GA RPE have problems with near vision in particular, even if it is retained subfoveal RPE central area. These problems are caused by paracentral scotomas, abnormal ability to adapt to the darkness that reduces visual acuity under dimmed lighting, and the deterioration of contrast sensitivity [31]. Magnifying aids paradoxically don't bring a large profit because it carries the magnified image into the paracentral absolute scotomas. The patient's vision during the day varies depending on the ability to find a central area functioning retina within the zone of GA [32].

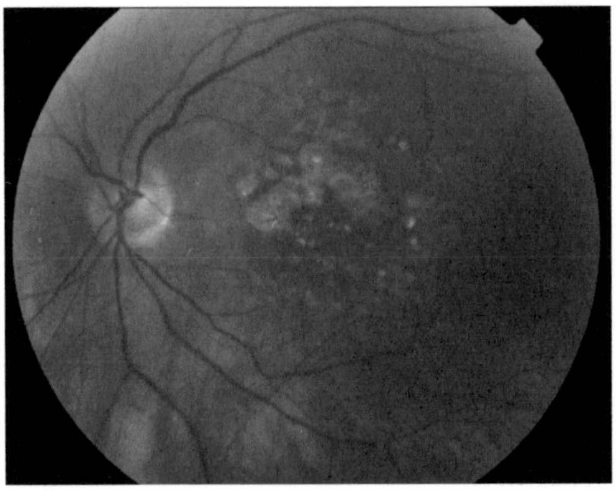

Figure 6. Geographic atrophy of RPE (red free image)

Long-term prognosis of visual acuity in GA is individual. It depends mainly on the location of the first location of GA. Interval from the developing of first spot to the GA with legal blindness is about 9 years [33]. The average rate of progress of GA is about 139 microns per year. Affected eyes have 8 % annual risk of a decline of visual acuity value from 20/50 to 20/100 [34].

GA RPE occurs bilaterally. The second eye is affected by in about 50%. Area of GA in the second eye is around 20 % smaller. With the development of GA in one eye decreases the risk of CNV in both eyes (i.e. wet AMD) [31].

Research that is based on the RPE injury hypothesis postulate that the pathogenesis and progression of dry macular degeneration is characterized by three distinct stages:

1. Initial RPE oxidant injury causes extrusion of cell membrane debris together with decreased activity of matrix metalloproteinases (MMPs), under the RPE as BLamD.

2. RPE cells are subsequently stimulated to increase synthesis of MMPs and other molecules responsible for extracellular matrix removal affecting both RPE basement membrane and BrM [35]. This process leads to progression of BLamD into BLinD and drusen

by admixture of blebs into BrM, followed by the formation of new basement membrane under the RPE to trap these deposits within BrM [36].

3. Macrophages are recruited to sites of RPE injury and deposit formation. Macrophage recruitment may be beneficial or harmful depending upon their activation status at the time of recruitment [37]. Nonactivated or scavenging macrophages may remove deposits without further injury. Activated or reparative macrophages, through the release of inflammatory mediators, growth factors, or other substances, may promote complications and progression to the late forms of the disease [37].

6.3. Wet form of AMD

Wet AMD occurs less commonly but is far more aggressive when compared with dry AMD. Wet AMD results from the development of neovascularization, or new blood vessel growth, beneath the retina. These abnormal blood vessels may break into the retinal cell layers. The leakage of fluid and proteins from these vessels causes scar formation throughout the macula, which ultimately results in deterioration of central vision. Wet AMD tends to be far more severe than dry AMD.

The wet form of AMD is characterized by occurrence of RPE detachment, choroidal neovascular membrane (CNV), subretinal hemorrhage in the macula. The terminal stage of wet AMD is disciform scar (Figure 7.).

In the last decade, the wet form of AMD allocated an additional 2 clinical units: angiomatose retinal proliferation (RAP) and polypoidal choroidal vasculopathy (PCV) (see below).

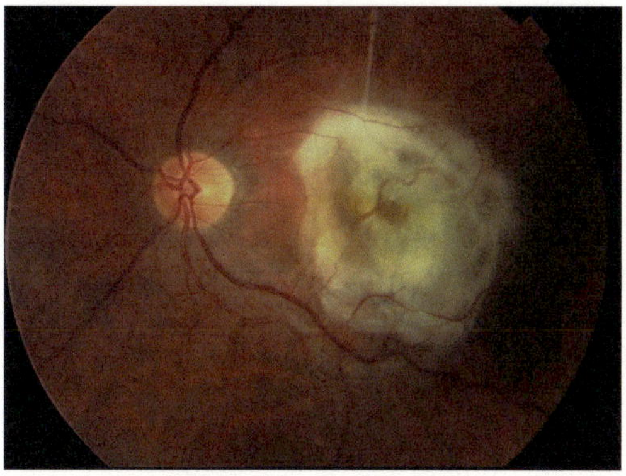

Figure 7. Disciform scar

Retinal pigment epithelium detachment

Their prognosis isn't good if central part of fovea is affected. [38]. RPE detachment is generally characterized by elevation of RPE layer from the Bruch's membrane. RPE detachment is divided into 4 categories.

1. Drusen RPE detachment (Figure 8.)

Drusen RPE detachment is formed in the later stages of multiple connecting soft drusen, which elevate the RPE layer from Bruch's membrane. Drusen RPE detachment is a high risk due to the development of CNV [38]. On the fluorescein angiography (FA) we can see in early phase hyperfluorescence of soft drusen, which isn't widening until the late stages.

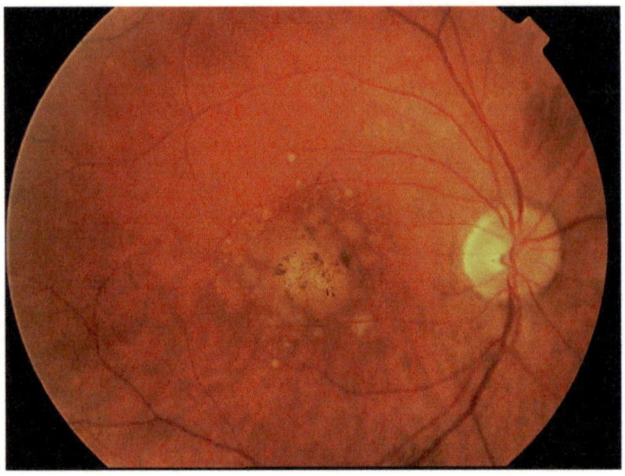

Figure 8. Drusen RPE detachment

2. Serous RPE detachment (Figure 9., Figure 10.)

Serous RPE detachment is roughly bounded elevation of the RPE cells, containing serous fluid that is usually clear, but may be turbid. On the FA we see early hyperfluorescence, which is sharply bounded, but not noticeable leakage.

3. Hemorrhagic RPE detachment (Figure 11.)

4. Fibrovascular RPE detachment (Figure 12.)

Hemorrhagic and vascularized RPE detachments are very close, because both contain the CNV. They differ from each other in principle, only the extent of bleeding, which in hemorrhagic RPE detachment greater. Angiographic picture of hemorrhagic RPE detachment is different from the vascularized because hemoglobin overlaps fluorescence, and the extent of CNV is not completely well defined. In unclear cases are possible to use indocyanine green angiography (ICGA), which can display the vascular structure of the retina and choroid despite hemoglobin.

The clinical course of RPE detachment may be as follows:

1. Persistent RPE detachment

Persistent RPE detachment can be stabilized without the presence of CNV. Over time, may be slowly progressing in its size [38].

2. Flattened RPE detachment

Flattening of the RPE detachment is uncommon and when it occurs, usually develops in the affected area geographic atrophy of the RPE [39].

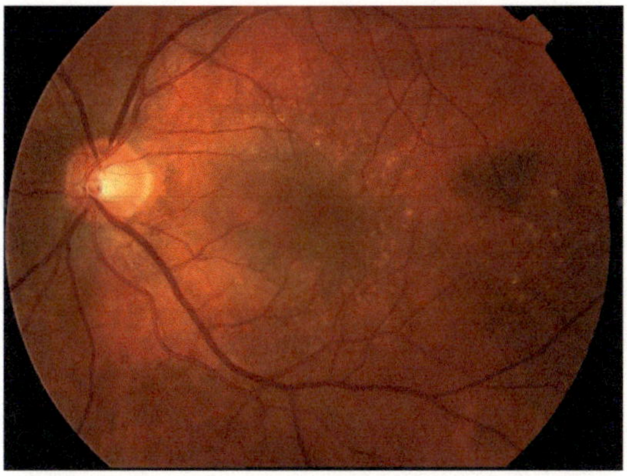

Figure 9. Serous RPE detachment

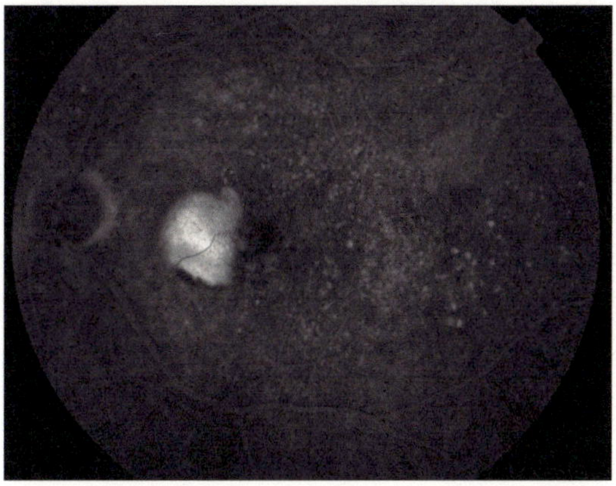

Figure 10. Serous RPE detachment on fluorescein angiography

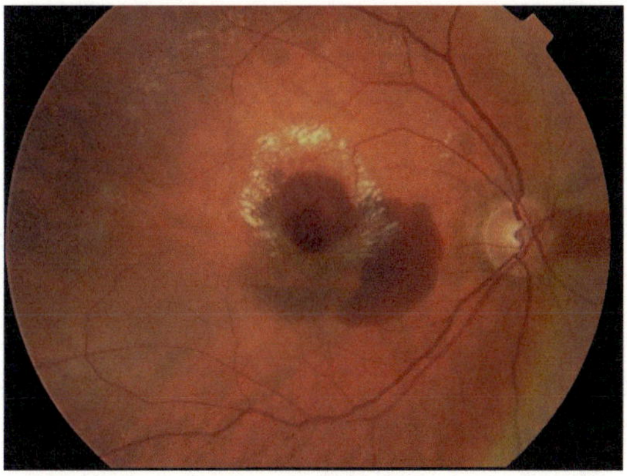

Figure 11. Hemorrhagic RPE detachment

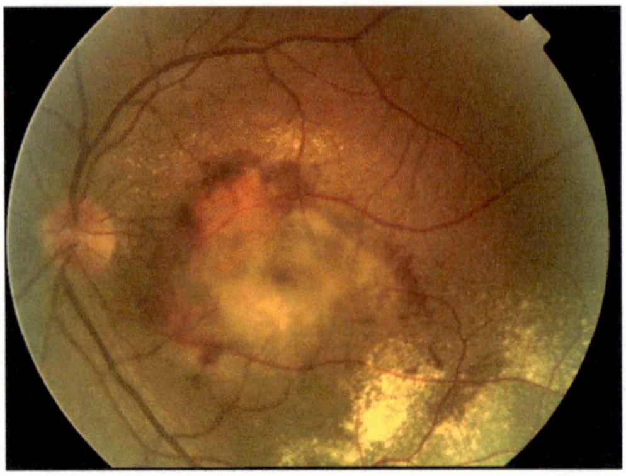

Figure 12. Fibrovascular RPE detachment

3. Rupture of RPE

RPE rupture is very unfavorable state accompanying the process of development of RPE detachment [40]. It occurs mostly at the edge of detachment at the transition attached and detached RPE. The RPE constricts away from location of rupture to the center of the detachment. If it is affected subfoveal area, there is detected a rapid decrease in visual acuity. In this case, the photoreceptors had lost contact with the RPE cells, and there is an absolute central scotoma. In the course of rupture usually occurs subretinal bleeding. Less frequently develops CNV, which is very aggressive and rapidly progresses to the disciform scar [40].

4. Development of CNV

But the most common complication of RPE detachment is the appearance of CNV. Increasing age is the basic risk factor of development of CNV in subjects with RPE detachment. CNV formation is rare in patients under 56 years of age, occurs in 29 % of those aged 56-75 years and affects 62.5 % of subjects in the group over 75 years. Another study showed that elderly patients have a larger RPE detachment with more fluid than younger and more often develop CNV [41].

Choroidal neovascular membrane

CNV occurs when occurs the rupture of Bruch's membrane. Newly formed blood vessels from choroid grow first into the space under the RPE and later under the subretinal space. Size of edema of neuroretina is a sign of CNV activity. Attempt to unify the classification of CNV has become a necessity. Based on this was defined by the term classic and occult CNV.

A typical picture of CNV includes subretinaly localized grayish lesion, which can vary in size, location and thickness. If the membrane has a classic character, the lesion is usually well defined and its edges are lined with subretinal hemorrhages (Figure 13.).

On the FA it can be seen from early stages well-demarcated lesion that not increase in it size to the late stages of FA (Figure 14., Figure 15.).

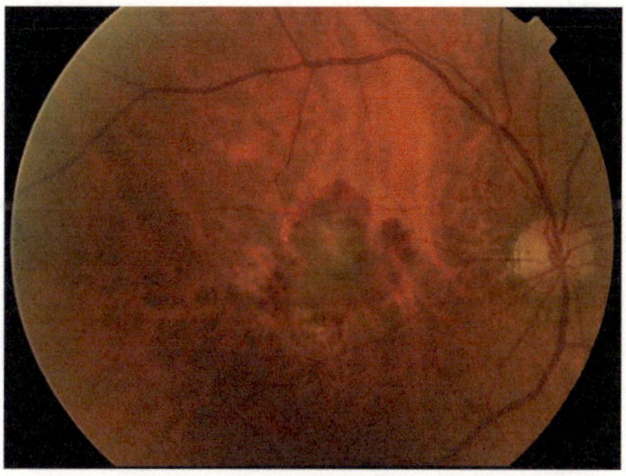

Figure 13. Classic CNV

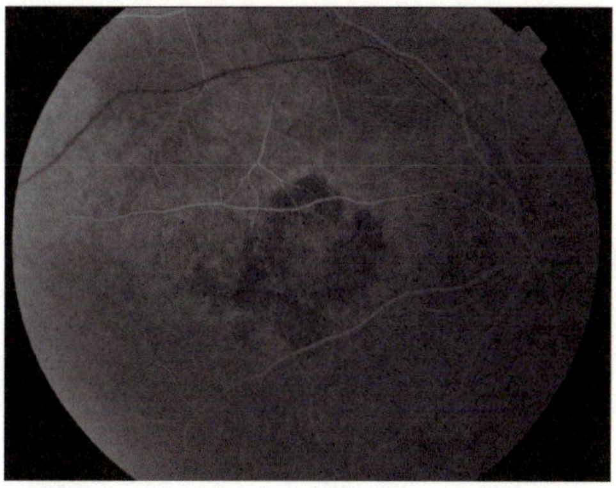

Figure 14. Early stage of classic CNV on FA, well-demarcated lesion with block of fluorescence on its border due to subretinal hemorrhage

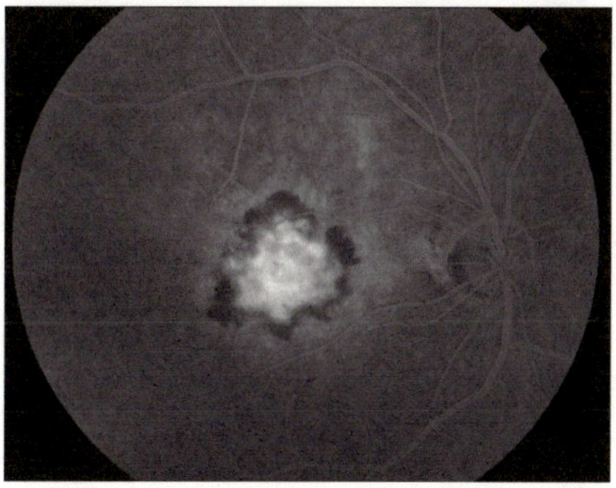

Figure 15. Late stage of classic CNV on FA, well-demarcated lesion that not increase in its size from early stage

The size of occult membranes is most evident at biomicroscopy. Changes are visible at the level of the RPE (movement of RPE cells, RPE detachment). There may occur subretinal hemorrhages. Oedema of neuroretina is noticeable (Figure 16.).

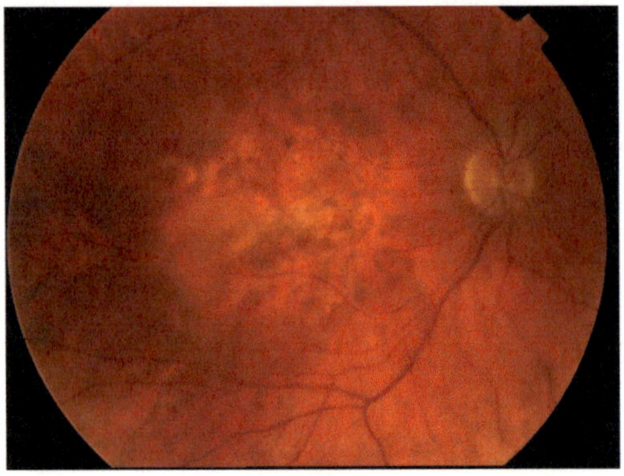

Figure 16. Occult CNV

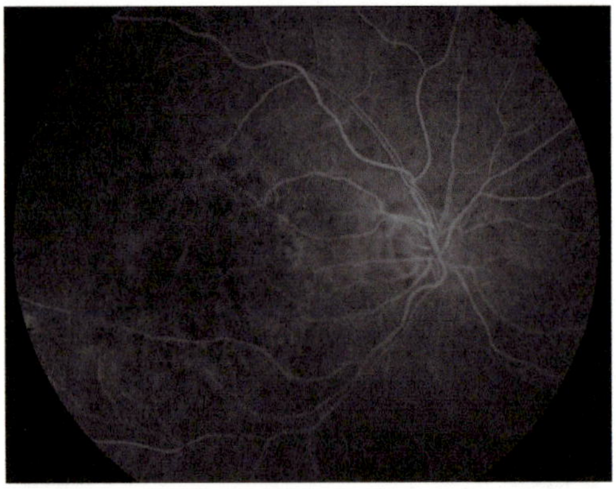

Figure 17. Early stage of occult CNV on FA, lesion is not clearly visible, leakage is very low and not well demarcated

Location of CNV in respect to the position of RPE

This classification is put into clinical practice for the first time in late 1960 by Gass [42].

Based on the findings on fluorescence angiography (FA) distinguishes two basic types of CNV: classic and occult.

Occult CNV (according to Gass classification type I) is characterized by the development of the neovascular complex and RPE choriocapillaris. CNV complex is characteristic for the beginning stages of wet AMD (Figures 16-18.).

http://dx.doi.org/10.5772/53762

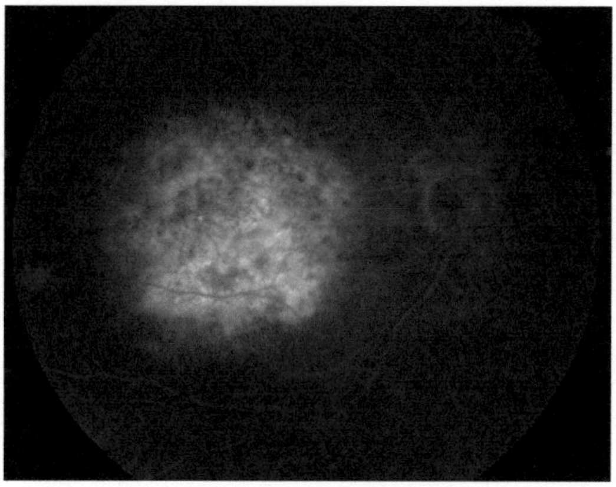

Figure 18. Late stage of occult CNV on FA, CNV size increases when compare to the early stage

Classic CNV (according to Gass classification type II) causes the spread of CNV complex in the space between the RPE and neuroretina. We can say that the classic CNV arises from occult CNV to a breach of continuity Bruch's membrane (Figures 13-15.).

Classification of CNV according to the center of the fovea

Entire CNV complex localization in respect to the center of the fovea plays a crucial role in deciding on the method of subsequent therapy. Localization is possible only by using of high-quality FA.

Depending on the position of CNV according to the fovea center we can diagnose 3 forms of CNV. The most common form is subfoveal localization, which has a CNV complex located beneath the center of the fovea. Another form is juxtafoveal localization. In this case, the CNV complex is located at a distance of 1 to 199 microns from the center of the fovea. The least frequent localization is extrafoveal location. Distance from the center of CNV complex fovea is larger than 200 microns.

Special clinical units within the wet form of AMD

In the last decades passed classification of wet AMD further development. There were created 2 new clinical entities distinguished from the model of classic and occult CNV: retinal angiomatous proliferation (RAP) and polypoidal choroidal vasculopathy (PCV).

Retinal Angiomatous Proliferation (RAP)

Yannuzzi created this term in order to describe the basic characteristics of clinical entity, in which the formation of neovascularization begins within retina [43].

RAP represents about 10 – 15 % of newly diagnosed cases of wet AMD [44]. It occurs more frequently in elderly patients [43]. Most commonly occurs in Caucasians, in contrast to PCV, which is more common in pigmented races [45].

The disease is divided into 3 clinical stages

Stage I – intraretinal neovascularization: New RAP lesions develop typically outside the foveal avascular zone, i.e. extrafoveal. The course is initially asymptomatic. Intraretinal neovascularization (IRN) begins in the deep capillary plexus outside the center of the fovea. During development, the most typically spread in the vertical direction, i.e. between the external and the internal limiting membrane. IRN that is spreading sideways is not typical in initial stages. Biomicroscopically can be observed capillary dilation with a large network of nourishing blood vessels and intraretinal haemorrhages. Haemorrhages are usually very discreet compared to subretinal hemorrhages accompanying classic and occult CNV and especially PCV [45].

Stage II - subretinal neovascularization: This stage is diagnosed if the complex of IRN moves between photoreceptors and RPE. This area develops detachment of neuroretina with corresponing edema. Intraretinal haemorrhages are more noticeable than in stage I. If the lesion extends into the subretinal space, there can be diagnosed small subretinal haemorrhage. At this stage, there is often retino-retinal anastomosis, which has afferent arteriole and efferent venule. Serous RPE detachment can be diagnosed if is IRN connected with subretinal CNV.

Stage III - CNV: In stage III is diagnosed already typical CNV combined with vascularized RPE detachment. During the development of CNV is then in subretinal space formed chorioretinal anastomosis like clear communication between the retinal bloodstream and the choriocapilaris. CNV is predominantly perfused by the vascular system of the choroid. In the end stage is then evident disciform scar.

Pathophysiological mechanism of RAP development is not explained in detail till now. It is assumed the proportion of VEGF produced by RPE cells [46]. Thus neovascularization begins intraretinally and later subretinally. Secondarily creates RPE detachment with the occult CNV [47]. Reduction of Bruch membrane permeability for VEGF may signify increases its intraretinal concentration. This situation is main cause of intraretinal neovascularization [48]. Another theory shows that the oxidative stress leads to migration of RPE cells, both subretinally and intraretinally. This leads to the production of VEGF and stimulation of neovascularization in an atypical location [49].

Diagnostic

Basic diagnostic modality is beside biomicroscopy FA examination. In stage I leakage occurs at the region intraretinal neovascularization. In this area is also biomicroscopicaly demonstrated edema with accumulation of vascular loops and leakage of dye on FA. RAP can at this stage be erroneously mistaken for another microangiopathy, such as incipient diabetic maculopathy. RAP stage II and I may be misdiagnosed as classic CNV. In stage III we can see on FA finding very close to vascularized RPE detachment. It is therefore often diagnosed as occult CNV [43].

ICGA usually brings enough light to the uncertain cases. In stage I is observed focal hyperfluorescence in retinal circulation, which has the character of IRN [44]. There can often be diagnosed retino-retinal anastomosis. In stage II IRN is visible inside and under the retina.

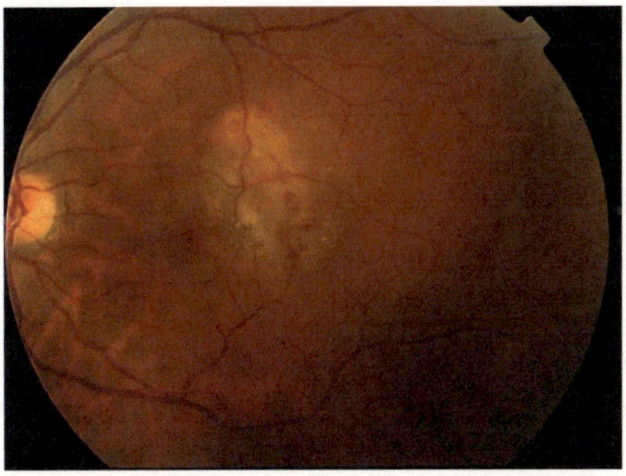

Figure 19. Stage III of RAP. Temporally in macula is chorioretinal anastomosis.

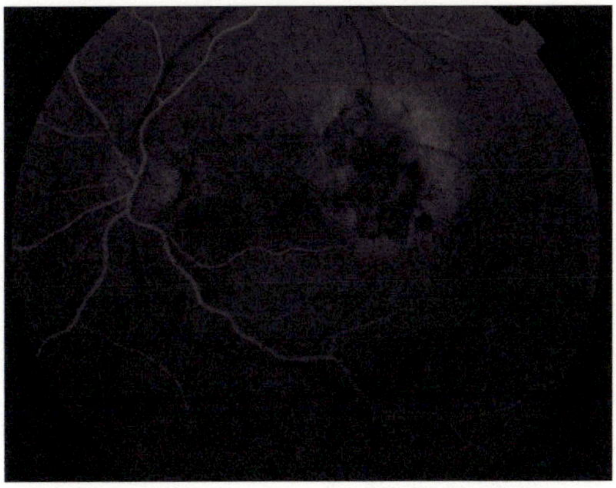

Figure 20. Stage III of RAP on FA, early phase

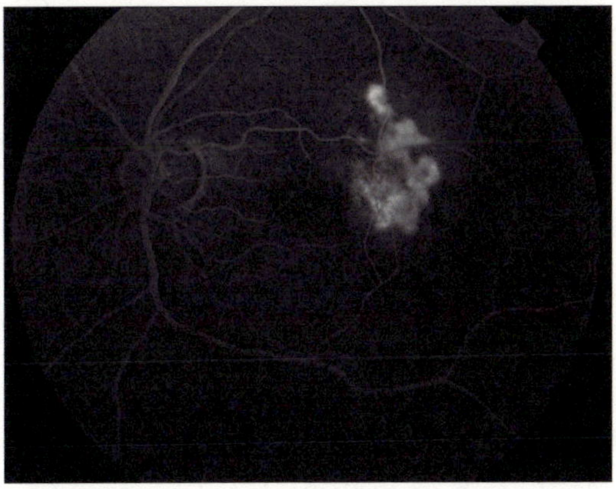

Figure 21. Stage III of RAP on FA, late phase, leakage dye from CNV is visible

For location of IRN have to be used pseudo stereo view to state the position of neovascularization in the vertical axis. Hot spot for RAP must be distinguished from another hot spots, e.g. inside the choroid. In stage III is visible, a connection of choroidal and retinal neovascularization (Figure 19.-21.). This creates a complex neovascularization, which has the character of vascularized RPE detachment. In some cases, we trace chorioretinal anastomosis.

Polypoidal Choroidal Vasculopathy (PCV)

This clinical entity has been in detail described and classified by Yannuzzi in 1990 as a peculiar hemorrhagic disorder of the macula, characterized by recurrent sub-retinal and sub-retinal pigment epithelium bleeding in middle aged black women [50]. Pathogenesis of the disease is not completely understood. The primary pathological changes that occur are sac-like extension of choroidal vessels, which are sacculated polypoidal nature. Clinically it is manifested by multiple hemorrhagic PCV and serose RPE detachment accompanied by retinal edema [50]. PCV is a special type of CNV in wet AMD [45].

PCV usually occurs in pigmented races between 50 - 65 years of age. Originally it was thought that the disease affected only black women. According to published data, the disease occurs in men, the ratio of affected women compared to men is 4,7:1 [51]. Prevalence varies between 4-10% in subjects with newly diagnosed wet AMD.

For the basic clinical picture of PCV is characterized by the absence drusen accompanied by haemorrhagic or serous RPE detachment. Other symptoms are: minimal signs of scarring, vitreous hemorrhage, and signs of intraocular inflammation. The disease usually occurs bilaterally [50], although it is described one-side occurrence [52]. The main factor contributing to the development of PCV seems to be the long-term chronic hypoxia by RPE detachment together with destructive effect of hard exudates.

Vascular structure PCV is located in choroid. Distinguish by size we have small, medium and large PCVs. PCV lesions reach a larger size if there are affected larger choroid vessels. When are affected medium choroid vessels, the lesions are smaller. Their diagnosis is more difficult because they don't have a characteristic image like a larger lesions [50].

PCV is located mostly around the optic disc. Some works but also show localization in the central periphery or in the central macular area [53]. PVC may be present as a single lesion, or may be multiple. Topographically are lesions localized to the area under the Bruch's membrane. The results of these studies are documented on OCT [54].

Natural course of the disease

PCV has the character of a chronic disease that manifests by serosanguinolent RPE detachment often near the optic nerve. Disease comes in multiple relapses, and patients have maintained good visual acuity for long time. Chronic RPE detachment usually results to the creation scaring plaque beneath the RPE, which is hardly distinguishable from classical disciform scar that develops as a terminal stage of the wet form of AMD. Polyps can have very specific progress. They occlude often spontaneously, and after some time are again perfunded. If are polyps located in the central subfoveal area in the terminal stage of the disease can occur RPE atrophy and chronic cystoid retinal changes. Rarely may arise massive subretinal and intravitreal hemorrhage, which is usually fatal and final visual acuity is poor [55].

Diagnostic

Blood vessels occurring with PCV have a characteristic shape. Form a bag-like aneurysms, RPE over them has a characteristic red-orange color (Figure 22., Figure 23.).

In contrast, blood vessels in other types of CNV are made from very small vascular knitting and are usually gray-green color. The thickness of the choroid is smaller in other types of CNVs. In PCV is choroid thicker.

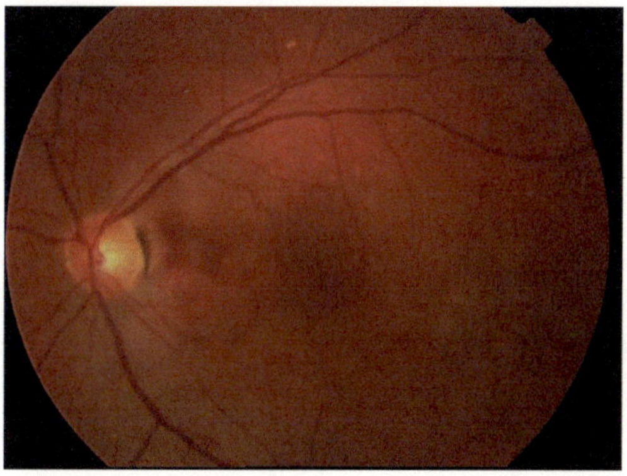

Figure 22. PCV in maculopapilar bundle, color image

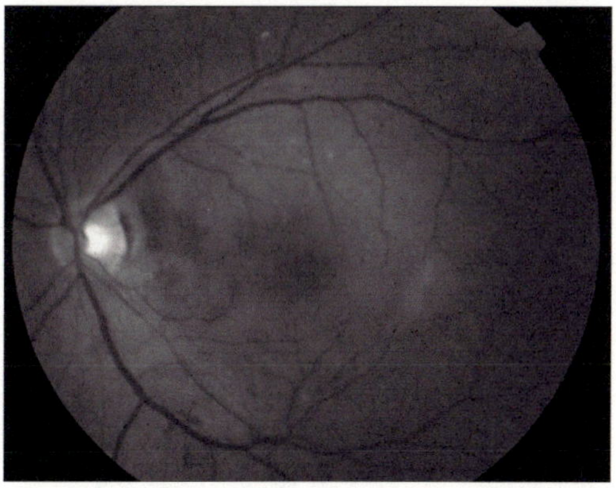

Figure 23. PCV in maculopapilar bundle, red free image

FA may in some cases provide a diagnosis of PCV (Figure 24., Figure 25.).

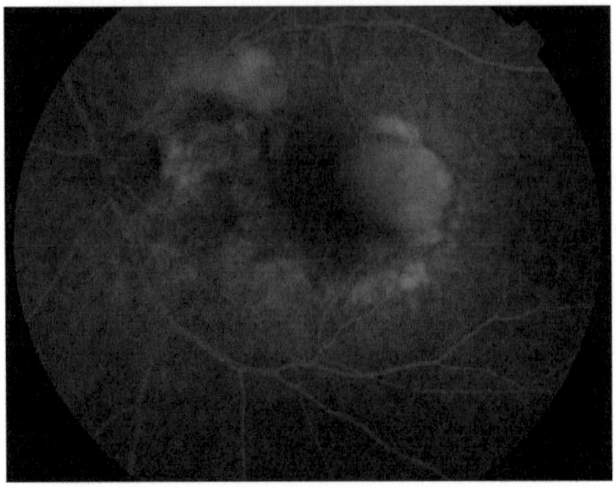

Figure 24. PCV in middle phase of FA, leakage from polyps is visible, in temporal part of macula is detected RPE detachment

However, the basic diagnostic modality is in the diagnosis of PVC ICGA. Only on ICGA can be diagnosed bag-like extension of choroidal vessels [56]. In the early phase of ICGA fill up large PCV vessel before filling of retinal vessels. Neighborhood of PCV lesions remains hypofluorescent. Late stage of ICGA shows choroidal polyps. They are closely associated with large chorioidal vessels (Figure 26., Figure 27.).

In the initial phase of the angiogram polyps are usually smaller than in the late phase. This corresponds to the red-orange lesions, which are detectable by biomicroscopy. In the late stage, there is a reverse phenomenon. Center of the lesion becomes hypofluorescent and around the polyp occurs hyperfluorescence. At a very late stage angiogram can occur washout of dye. This phenomenon is only seen in the lesions without leaking; leaking lesions remain hyperfluorescent [56].

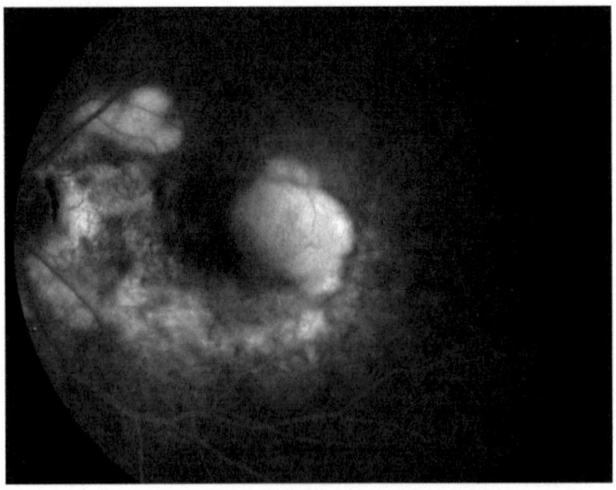

Figure 25. PCV in late phase of FA, leakage from polyps is visible, 2 RPE detachments are located on temporal upper vascular arcade and in temporal part of macula

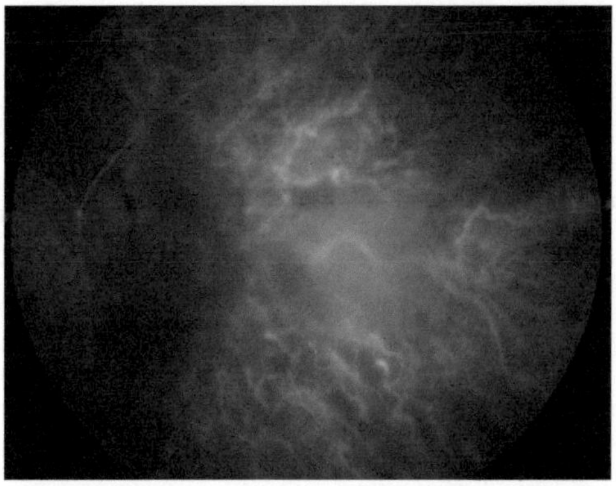

Figure 26. PVC, early stage on ICGA

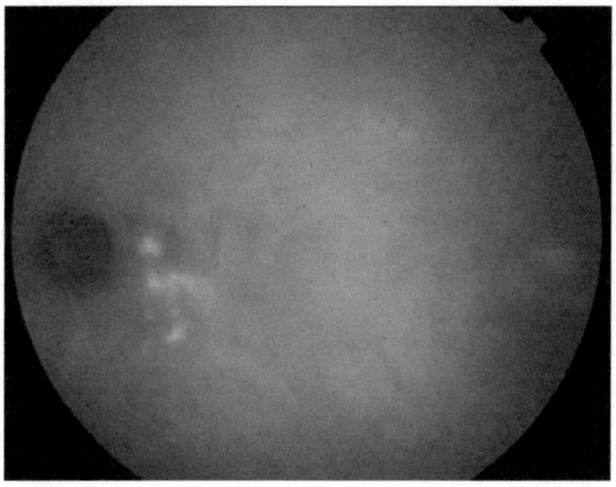

Figure 27. PCV, late stage on ICGA, polyps are visible near the optic disc

OCT examination demonstrates elevation of RPE layer, which corresponds to the red-orange lesions detected during biomicroscopic examination. PCV is manifested against serous RPE ablation by greater prominence of RPE layer [54].

Differential diagnosis

Differential diagnosis distinguishes PCV from other vascular abnormalities, inflammatory conditions of the retina and choroid, other types of CNV and choroidal tumors. Improved diagnostic methods and clarifying the pathophysiological mechanisms lead to the correct diagnosis of PCV more often than before.

In diagnostic help both FA and ICGA. CNV in PCV leaks already at an early phase, so as CNV different origin. In the late stage, the lesion on the basis of PVC may have washed out the dye [56]. If a bag-like aneurysms leak, in their neighborhood is evident late dye leakage (Figure 26., Figure 27.).

CNV on the basis of PVC, rarely undergo to fibrose unlike other types of CNV in AMD. RPE detachment associated with PCV almost doesn't fibrose, whereas RPE detachment associated with occult CNV fibrose very often and has a very poor prognosis [50].

Author details

Petr Kolar

Address all correspondence to: pe-kolar@seznam.cz

Department of Ophthalmology, University Hospital Brno and Masaryk University Brno, Czech Republic

References

[1] De Jong P T V M. Age-related Macular Degeneration. The New England Journal of Medicine. 2006; 355(14), 1474-85.

[2] Lim L S, Mitchell P, Seddon J M, Johanna M et al. Ophthalmology 1: Age-related Macular Degeneration. Lancet. 2012; 379, 1728-1738.

[3] Smith W, Assink J, Klein R, et al. Risk factors for age-related macular degeneration: Pooled findings from three continents. Ophthalmology. 2001; 108, 697-704.

[4] Friedman D S, Katz J, Bressler N M, Rahmani B, Tielsch JM. Racial differences in the prevalence of age-related macular degeneration: the Baltimore Eye Survey. Ophthalmology. 1999; 106, 1049-55.

[5] Laude A, Cackett P D, Vithana E N, et al. Polypoidal choroidal vasculopathy and neovascular age-related macular degeneration: same or different disease? Prog Retin Eye Res. 2010; 29 19-29.

[6] Gupta B, Jyothi S, Sivaprasad S. Current treatment options for retinal angiomatous proliferans (RAP). Br J Ophthalmol. 2010; 94, 672-77.

[7] Klein R, Klein B E, Knudtson M D, Meuer S M, Swift M, Gangnon R E. Fifteen-year cumulative incidence of age-related macular degeneration: the Beaver Dam Eye Study. Ophthalmology. 2007; 114, 253-62.

[8] Seddon J M, Willett W C, Speizer F E, Hankinson S E. A prospective study of cigarette smoking and age-related macular degeneration in women. JAMA. 1996; 276, 1141-46.

[9] Seddon J M, Cote J, Davis N, Rosner B. Progression of age-related macular degeneration: association with body mass index, waist circumference, and waist-hip ratio. Arch Ophthalmol, 2003; 121, 785-92.

[10] Chakravarthy U, Wong TY, Fletcher A, et al. Clinical risk factors for age-related macular degeneration: a systematic review and meta-analysis. BMC Ophthalmol. 2010; 10, 31.

[11] Snow KK, Seddon JM. Do age-related macular degeneration and cardiovascular disease share common antecedents? Ophthalmic Epidemiol. 1999; 6, 125-43.

[12] Chew E Y, Sperduto R D, Milton R C, et al. Risk of advanced age-related macular degeneration after cataract surgery in the Age-Related Eye Disease Study: AREDS report 25. Ophthalmology. 2009; 116, 297-303.

[13] McKay G J, Patterson C C, Chakravarthy U, et al. Evidence of association of APOE with age-related macular degeneration- a pooled analysis of 15 studies. Hum Mutat. 2011; 32, 1407-16.

[14] Yu Y, Bhangale TR, Fagerness J, et al. Common variants near FRK/ COL10A1 and VEGFA are associated with advanced age-related macular degeneration. Hum Mol Genet. 2011; 20, 3699-709.

[15] Laatikainen L, Karinkari J. Capillary-free area of the fovea with advancing age. Invest Ophthalmol Vis Sci. 1977; 161, 1154-1157.

[16] Klein R, Klein B E K, Linton K L P. Prevalence of age-related maculopathy: the Beaver Dam Eye Study. Ophthalmology. 1992; 99, 933-943.

[17] Groh M J M, Michelson G, Langhans M J, et al. Influence of age on retinal and optic nerve head blood circulation. Ophthalmology. 1996; 103, 529-534.

[18] Ibrahim Y W M, Bots M L, Mulder P G H, et al. Number of perifoveolar vessels in aging, hypertension, and atherosclerosis: the Rotterdam Study. Invest Ophthalmol Vis Sci. 1998; 39,1049-53.

[19] Gao H, Hollyfield J G. Aging of the human retina: differential loss of neurons and retinal pigment epithelial cells. Invest Ophthalmol Vis Sci. 1992; 33, 1-17.

[20] Sanberg M A, Gaudio, A R. Slow photostress recovery and disease severity in age-related macular degeneration. Retina. 1995; 15, 407-412.

[21] Grunwald J E, Hariprasad S M, Dupont J, et al. Foveolar choroidal blood flow in age-related macular degeneration. Invest Ophthalmol Vis Sci. 1998; 39, 385-390.

[22] Curcio C A, Saunders P L, Younger P W, et al. Peripapillary chorioretinal atrophy: Bruch's membrane changes and photoreceptor loss. Ophthalmology. 2000; 107, 334-343.

[23] Hazin R, Freeman P, David M D, Kahook M Y. Age- Related Macular Degeneration: A Guide for the Primary Care Physician. Journal of the National Medical Association. 2009; 101, 134-138.

[24] Noble J, Chaudhary V. Age-related Macular Degeneration. Canadian Medical Asscia-tion Jornal. 2010; 16, 1759.

[25] Mettu P S, Wielgus A R, Ong S S, Cousins S W. Retinal pigment epithelium response to oxidant injury in the pathogenesis of early age-related macular degeneration. Molecular Aspects of Medicine. 2012; 33, 376-398.

[26] D'Souza Y, Jones C J P, Bonshek R. Glycoproteins of drusen and drusen-like lesions. J Mol Hist. 2008; 39, 77-86.

[27] Kliffen M, van der Schaft T L, Mooy C M, de Jong P T. Morphologic changes in age-related maculopathy. Microscopy Research and Technique. 1997; 36 (2), 106–122.

[28] Green, W R. Histopathology of age-related macular degeneration. Molecular vision. 1999; 5, 27.

[29] Penfold P L, Madigan M C, Gillies M C, Provis J M. Immunological and aetiological aspects of macular degeneration. Progress in Retinal and Eye Research. 2001; 20 (3), 385–414.

[30] Fine S L, Berger J W, Maguire M G, et al. Age related macular degeneration. N Engl J Med. 2000; 342, 483-492.

[31] Sunness J S, Rubin G S, Applegate C A, et al. Visual function abnormalities and prognosis in eyes with age-related geographic atrophy of the macula and the good visual acuity. Ophthalmology. 1997; 104, 1677-1691.

[32] Sunness J S, Gonzales-Baron J, Applegate C A, et al. Enlargement of atrophy and visual acuity loss in the geographic atrophy form of age-related macular degeneration. Ophthalmology. 1999; 106, 1768-1779.

[33] Maguire P, Vine A K. Geographic atrophy of retinal pigment epithelium. Am J Ophthalmol. 1986; 102, 621-625.

[34] Schatz H, McDonald H R. Atrophic macular degeneration: rate of spread of geographic atrophy and visual loss. Ophthalmology. 1989; 96, 1541-1551.

[35] Strunnikova N, Zhang C, Teichberg D, Cousins S W, Baffi J, Becker K G, Csaky K G. Survival of retinal pigment epithelium after exposure to prolonged oxidative injury: a detailed gene expression and cellular analysis. Investigative Ophthalmology and Visual Science. 2004; 45 (10), 3767–3777.

[36] Espinosa-Heidmann D G, Suner I J, Catanuto P, Hernandez E P, Marin-Castano M E, Cousins S W. Cigarette smoke-related oxidants and the development of sub-RPE deposits in an experimental animal model of dry AMD. Investigative Ophthalmology and Visual Science. 2006; 47 (2), 729–737.

[37] Cousins S W, Espinosa-Heidmann D G, Csaky K G. Monocyte activation in patients with age-related macular degeneration: a biomarker of risk for choroidal neovascularization? Archives of Ophthalmology. 2004; 122 (7), 1013–1018.

[38] Casswell A G, Kohen D, Bird,A C. Retinal pigment epithelial detachment in the elderly: classification and outcome. Br J Ophthalmol. 1985; 69, p. 379-403.

[39] Blair C J. Geographic atrophy of retinal pigment epithelium. Arch Ophthalmol. 1975; 93. 19-25.

[40] Green S N, Yarian D. Acute tear of the retinal pigment epithelium. Retina. 1983; 3, 16-20.

[41] Yannuzzi L A, Gitter K A, Schatz H. Detachment of the retinal pigment epithelium. In: The Macula: A Comprehensive Text and Atlas. Baltimore: Williams and Wilkins; 1979, 166-179.

[42] Gass J D M. Pathogenesis of disciform detachment of neuroepithelium III. Senile disciform macular degeneration. Am J Ophthalmol. 1967; 63, 617-644.

[43] Yannuzzi L A, Negrao S, Iida T et al. Retinal angiomatous proliferation in the age-related macular degeneration. Retina. 2001; 21, 416-434.

[44] Lafaut B A, Aisenbrey S, Broecke C V, et al. Clinicopathological correlation of deep retinal vascular anomalous complex in age-related macular degeneration. Br J Ophthalmol. 2000; 84, p. 1268-1274.

[45] Yannuzzi L A, Wong D W K, Sforzolino B S, et al. Polypoidal choroidal vasculopathy and neovascularized age-related macular degeneration. Arch Ophthalmol. 1999; 117, 1503- 1510.

[46] Wells J A, Murthy R, Chibber R, et al. Levels of vascular endothelial growth factor are elvated in the vitreous in patients with subretinal neovascularization. Br J Ophthalmol. 1996; 363-366.

[47] Tobe T, Okamoto N, Vinores M A, et al. Evolution of neovascularization in mice with overexpression of vascular endothelial growth factor in photoreceptor. Invest Ophthalmol Vis Sci. 1998; 39, p. 180-188.

[48] Khiffen M, Sharma H S, Moory C M, et al. Increased expression of angiogenic growth factors in age-related maculopathy. Br J Ophthalmol. 1997; 81, 1154-1162.

[49] Tamai K, Spaide R F, Ellis E A, et al. Lipid hydroperoxide-stimulated subretinal choroidal neovascularization in the rabbit. Exp Eye Res. 2002; 74, 301-308.

[50] Yannuzzi L A, Sorenson J, Spaide R F, et al. Idiopathic polypoidal choroidal vasculopathy. Retina. 1990; 10, 1-8.

[51] Uayma M, Wada M, Nagai Y, et al. Polypoidal choroidal vasculopathy: natural history. Am J Ophthalmol. 2002; 133, 639-648.

[52] Iida T, Yannuzzi L A, Freund K B, et al. Retinal angiopathy and polypoidal choroidal vasculopathy. Retina. 2002; 22, 455-463.

[53] Yannuzzi L A, Nogueira F B, Spaide R F, et al. Idiopathic polypoidal choroidal vasculopathy: a peripheral lesions. Arch Ophthalmol. 1998; 116, p. 382-383.

[54] Iijima H, Iida T, Imai M, et al. Optical coherence tomography of orange-red subretinal lesions in eyes with idiopathic polypoidal vasculopathy. Am J Ophthalmol. 2000; 129, 105- 111.

[55] Yang S S, Fu A D, McDonald H R, et al. Massive spontaneous choroidal hemorrhage. Retina. 2003; 23, 139-144.

[56] Spaide R F, Yannuzzi L A, Slakter J S, et al. Indocyanine green videoangiography of idiopathic polypoidal choroidal vasculopathy. Retina. 1995; 15, 100-110.

Chapter 4

New Insights into the Optical Coherence Tomography – Assessement and Follow-Up of Age-Related Macular Degeneration

Simona-Delia Ţălu

Additional information is available at the end of the chapter

http://dx.doi.org/10.5772/53357

1. Introduction

Optical coherence tomography (OCT) is a relatively new noninvasive optical imaging method that has revolutionized the way we see the retina. It uses near-infrared light in order to deliver high-resolution cross-sectional images of the macula that are very similar to the histopathological specimens. However, the OCT images are not the direct depiction of the anatomical structures, but they represent the consequence of the optical properties of the tissues being scanned [1]. The retinal microarchitecture can be visualized as cross-sectional or tomographic volumetric data. The OCT has been used increasingly over the past several years to diagnose and monitor a variety of retinal diseases that affect the macula. Age – related Macular Degeneration (AMD) is one of the retinal diseases that benefited the most from the development of OCT techniques. In the exudative form of the disease, OCT identifies intraretinal fluid and outlines the choroidal neovascularization. However, it is not able to resolve the internal structure of the fibro-vascular membranes, as it cannot distinguish very clearly between their various components: new vessels, fibrous tissue, blood, dense exudates. OCT is extremely useful in the management and monitoring of wet AMD: it allows early diagnosis and helps in the decision-making process of retreatment with anti-VEGF agents [2]. OCT became an indispensable tool in the diagnosis of neovascular recurrences by identifying fluid under or in the retina [3]. Newer spectral domain OCT devices permit the detailed description of drusens in early AMD that allows the refined phenotyping of the disease [2]. By allowing detailed description of various lesions in AMD, OCT is bringing significant contributions for progressing in the understanding of AMD pathogenesis.

2. Problem statement

A variety of retinal diseases such as AMD, central serous chorio-retinopathy, macular hole, vitreo-macular interface syndrome and diabetic maculopathy have taken advantage from the introduction of OCT in the clinical practice. Among these, AMD is the ocular condition that benefited the most from the enormous advantages offered by OCT imaging techniques, in terms of diagnosis, response to treatment and monitoring. Future progress in OCT techniques has already brought and is expected to bring new insights in understanding the pathophysiology of this potentially blinding disease. With the aim of defining the role of OCT in the assessment and follow up of AMD, the theoretical principles at the foundation of this retinal imaging technique are outlined, making a clear distinction between TD-OCT and SD-OCT methods. The advantages of SD-OCT over TD-OCT methods are revealed. The role of OCT in AMD management is emphasized by the description of typical OCT aspects in various AMD lesions: macular edema, CNV membranes, occult and classic choroidal neovascularization, pigment epithelial detachments (PED), external retinal cysts, vitreo-macular adhesions. OCT has a crucial role in monitoring AMD and establishing the indication of treatment with anti-VEGF intravitreal injections in the wet form of the disease. The place of OCT in the evaluation of AMD patients is completed by its comparative presentation with retinal biomicroscopy, fluorescein and indocyanine green angiography. The impact of OCT in AMD diagnosis and monitoring is illustrated with examples of various aspects that AMD can display, both with a TD-OCT device (Stratus OCT) and a SD-OCT one (Cirrus OCT). Future directions in OCT techniques development close the current presentation.

3. Theoretical considerations on OCT examination techniques

3.1. History

The concept of optical coherence tomography (OCT) was developed at Massachusetts Institute of Technology in the early 1990s and the first commercial version of OCT was made available by Carl Zeiss (Jena, Germany) in 1996 [4]. The first applications of OCT were to provide quantitative and qualitative information about the peripapillary area of the retina and the coronary artery [5]. The first publication on time-domain OCT belongs to Huang and coworkers in 1991 [5]. Hee et al. published the first data on the quantitative evaluation of the macular edema in 1995 [6]. Since its introduction, OCT evolved into a powerful examination tool for patients with retinal diseases [7].

3.2. Optical tomography versus ultrasound

For many years, the cross-sectional imaging of the eye has been possible only with the help of ultrasounds which allowed spatial resoultions of 150 μm. The development of new techniques was based on the use of higher frequency waves that created the possibility to obtain image resolutions of 20 μm. However, the strong atenuation in the biological tissues limits its use to the anterior structures of the eye [8]. The principles of the two imaging methods

(OCT and ultrasounds) are similar, but OCT uses light instead of sound. The primary difference between ultrasonic and optical imaging derivates from the different speed of sound and light. The light propagates nearly a million of times faster than sound, which allows the obtaining of measurements resolutions in the range of 10 μm or less at the posterior pole of the eye. Also, the use of light makes the examination more comfortable for the patient, as there is no need for physical contact with the examined eye [8].

3.3. OCT Instrumentation for retinal imaging

The device operates as a fundus camera: a condensing lens of +78 dioptres is used so that the retina could be imaged in the same plane with the instrument. The magnification of the retinal image is determined by two factors: the refractive power of the condensing lens and the magnification of the ocular. At the lowest magnification, the typical field of view is 30º. If the visual acuity of the eye to be examined is very low and therefore the patient has fixation problems, a guiding light can be placed in front of the fellow eye, in order to stabilize the eyes during image acquisition. With the first generation OCT devices, pupil dilation was recommended with the aim of obtaining high quality images, but the latest generation OCT machines deliver good quality pictures with a 3-mm diameter pupil. The OCT technology can be limited by various conditions of the eye: lens or vitreal opacities, subretinal haemorrhages, lack of foveal fixation, nystagmus [8].

3.4. Principle of OCT

OCT is based on the interferometry that uses a low-coherence light in order to measure the difference between the reflected light waves from the examined tissue and that from a reference path [9]. The light reflected from the retinal structures interferes with the light of the reference beam. The detection of echoes resulting from this interference is measuring the light echoes versus depth [9,10].

Axial resolution. Axial resolution is given by the bandwdith of the light source and the level of coherence that depends upon the central wavelength [10]. The light from a superluminiscent diode has long coherence that generates images with poor axial resolution. With short-coherence light, interference is possible over short distances and therefore high axial resolution is possible [10].

Transverse resolution. The transverse resolution is determined by the size of the light spot that can be focused on the retina. The best structural resolution is obtained when the light is focused on the tissue to be examined. The absorbtion of central light by the tissue of interest must also be considered [10].

3.5. Time Domain (TD-OCT) versus Spectral Domain (SD-OCT)

OCT is applied by two main methods: TD-OCT and SD-OCT.

TD-OCT produces two-dimensional images of the sample internal structure. An A-scan represents a reflectivity profile in depth which is gradually built up over time by moving a mirror in the reference arm of the interferometer. A B-scan depicts a cross-section image meaning a lateral x depth map which is generated by collecting many A-scans [4].

SD-OCT can be implemented in two formats, Fourier domain (FD-OCT) and swept source (SS-OCT). With SD-OCT units, all the A-scans in the reflected light are acquired at a given point in tissue. The moving mirror is not needed in order to obtain complete A-scans which allows the acquisition of the images about 60 times faster than with TD-OCT. The detection and monitoring of retinal diseases is improved with SD-OCT units because they have ultra high-speed scan rate, superior axial and lateral resolution, cross-sectional (2D) scan, 3D raster scanning and a higher imaging sensitivity than the traditional TD-OCT units. The SD-OCT software is much improved compared with traditional TD-OCT and the great number of scans done per unit of time creates the conditions for the SD-OCT systems to generate 3D reconstructions which can be further manipulated with the aim to demonstrate subtle pathology not evident with conventional 2D images [4].

Briefly, the advantages of SD-OCT over TD-OCT are: significant improvement of the image axial resolution, decreased acquisition times, reduction of motion artifacts, increased area of retinal sampling and the possibility to create topographic maps by the three-dimensional evaluation of tissues [11,12].

Table 1 summarizes the main differences between TD-OCT and SD-OCT.

Property	TD-OCT	SD-OCT
Principle	Low coherence interferometry	Fourier transformation
Modality of acquisition	An interferometer measures **sequentially** the echo delay time of light that is reflected by the retinal microstructures	A spectrometer evaluates **simultaneously** the light reflection by the retinal microstructures
Modality of sampling	It samples one point at the time	It samples all the points simultaneously
Image acquisition time	1 – 2 seconds	60 times faster
Sampled area	6 radial scans are performed, 20 μ wide and 6 mm long (the area between the 6 scans is not imaged)	In a 6-mm diameter area, 65.000 scans are performed, without excluding areas; 128-200 scans over the same area
Rate of acquisition	Cross-section images of the retina are obtained every 1.6 seconds: 400 scans/second	25.000 – 52.000 scans/second
Presentation of the results	Two-dimensional images of the sample internal structure	3D reconstruction possible
Image axial resolution	10 - 15 μm	3-7 μm

Table 1. The main differences between the properties of TD-OCT and SD-OCT

4. TD-OCT

4.1. Principle of TD-OCT

The origin of TD-OCT imaging technique is found in the processes of absorbtion and dispersion of light traversing tissues [13]. The creation of an image with the TD-OCT technique is based on the principle of *low coherence interferometry*. The source of light is represented by a superluminiscent diode that emits a radiation with the wavelength of 830-840 nm. This emission is split in two arms by an optical beam splitter functioning as interferometer: half the beam is reflected from the reference mirror and is named the *reference beam* and half of it is directed to the target tissue and is named the *detection beam*. The comparison of the tissue-reflected beam with the beam coming from the reference mirror measures the time delay between these two beams [13]. In order to understand the system operating, the corpuscular theory of light must be applied: the beam is made up of short pulses of light. The pulse of light reflected from the reference mirror and the pulse of light coming from the analyzed tissue within the eye will coincide only if they both arrive at the same time, producing the phenomenon called *light interference*. For the light interference to occur, the distance traveled by the two above mentioned beams must be equal. The interference is measured by a light-sensitive detector and it is translated into OCT image on the screen [8]. This method allowed to obtain cross-section images of the retina every 1.6 seconds (400 A-scans per second) [14]. TD-OCT has limits represented by: long acquisition times, limited image sampling (with the risk of overlooking small macular lesions), limited resolution by motion artifacts and patient blinking [14].

4.2. Tomographic imaging and volumetry – Interpretation of TD-OCT images

The light source moves across the retina and the optical reflection and backscatter from the retinal structures are detected. Successive longitudinal measurements at transversal sequential points are performed. This technique generates a two-dimensional image and a cross-sectional map displayed in false colours. Each colour is given a certain degree of reflectivity. White and red colours corespnd to highly reflective tissues, whereas black and blue represent low reflectivity structures. Green is given an intermediate reflectivity. Examples of hyperreflective tissues are: fibrosis, haemorrhages, infiltrates [8]. The retinal layers are displayed on the linear scans and the retinal thickness can be measured taking as references the vitreo-retinal interface and the retinal pigmented epithelium, given their different reflectivity. By using 6 radial scans 30 degrees apart, a surface map can be obtained, in which white and red represent high volume structures (for example, macular edema) and black and blue correspond to thinned retinal areas [8].

4.3. Image resolution

The most important parameter that determines OCT image resolution is the coherence length of the light source. For the commercially available TD-OCT system, image axial resolution is in the range of 10-15 μm. The penetration through transparent optical media is excellent, but through a thick haemorrhage is less than 100 μm [8].

4.4. Image processing and correction for eye motions

Image acquisition takes about 1-2 seconds. Taking into account that the image resolution is extremely high, the correction for eye motions is very important to avoid the obtaining of blurred images. As consequence, image processing techniques had to be developed [8].

5. SD-OCT

5.1. Principle of SD-OCT

The development of the SD-OCT technique is originating in the Fourier mathematical equation (1807). The french mathematician Joseph Fourier described the decomposition of a periodic function into a sum of simple sinusoidal-based oscillating functions. The practical effect of this abstract statement is the possibility to measure simultaneously all echoes of light, in contrast to TD-OCT where the echoes of light are measured sequentially by moving a mirror in front of the reference beam. The SD-OCT devices use a central wavelength of 800-850 nm, a stationary reference arm, a high speed spectrometer that analyses simultaneously all the frequencies and a charged-coupled device (CCD) line-scan camera. The mechanical scanning is not needed in order to detect light echoes simultaneously. As consequence, the aquisition speed increases to 25,000-52,000 A-scan/second and the amount of data that can be obtained during one session was improved significantly [15]. The axial resolution is of 3-7 μm (as compared to 10 – 15 μm with TD-OCT devices), significantly improving the signal-to-noise ratio. Therefore, the detection of individual retinal layers and lesions components became possible [16].

5.2. Clinical impact of SD-OCT

The practical impact of the improvement in axial image resolution is the early detection of small cystic changes associated with the wet form of AMD. The early diagnosis is very important for the early treatment and the better preservation of the visual function. Given the possibility to get images simultaneously in various planes, the 3D reconstruction is possible with SD-OCT, allowing the obtaining of hundreds of high-resolution images per second and the accurate measurement of the macula (total volume) in various conditions: edema, fluid, drusen, CNV. The reduction of the examination time considerably decreases the artifacts related to eye movements and poor fixation of the low vision patients [17]. Another significant advantage of SD-OCT is represented by the increased retinal scan coverage. The SD-OCT images have proven to be clearer and with higher quality as compared to the ones obtained by the successive TD-OCT systems (OCT1, OCT3, stratus). The SD-OCT systems are continuously improving, by adding complementary functions: fundus photography, angiography, microperimetry. The ultra-high resolution images obtained by SD-OCT allow a better differentiation between the retinal and subretinal layers [4].

5.3. Commercially available SD-OCT devices

SD-OCT has superior depth resolution as compared to TD-OCT. Currently, the axial resolution varies from 3 – 7 μm, depending on the SD-OCT model [18]. Several SD-OCT instruments are available at the current moment: Cirrus HD-OCT (Carl Zeiss Meditec), RTVue-Fourier DomainOCT (Optovue), Copernicus OCT (Reichert/-Optopol Technology), Spectral OCT/SLO (Opko/Oti), Spectralis HRA+OCT (Heidelberg Engineering), Topcon 3D OCT-1000 (Topcon) and RS-3000 Retiscan (Nidek). All the above mentioned instruments provide high quality images and offer the possibility of tridimensional reconstruction of the macula [13]. The main technical characteristics and differences between the commercially available SD-OCT devices are presented in table 2 [15].

Device (Company)	Axial resolution (μm)	A-scans/second
Cirrus HD-OCT (Carl Zeiss Meditec)	5	27 000
Spectralis (Heidelberg Engineering)	7	40 000
RTVue-100 (Optovue)	5	26 000
3D-OCT 1000 3D-OCT 2000 (Topcon)	6	18 000
Spectral OCT/SLO (OPKO/OTI)	5	27 000
SOCT Copernicus (Optopol)	6	25 000
SOCT Copernicus HR (Canon/Optopol, Inc)	3	50 000
SDOCT (Bioptigen)	4	20 000
Retinascan RS-3000 (Nidek)	7	53 000

Table 2. Commercially available SD-OCT devices

6. Application area of OCT in AMD

6.1. Overview

Most cases of neovascular AMD are complicated by intraretinal fluid accumulation and RPE detachments. For many years, the therapeutic decision in neovascular AMD was based on the results of fundus biomicroscopy, fluorescein and indocyanine green angiography. In this context, the posttherapeutical evolution in many CNV membranes remained unsatisfactory. OCT technology offers subtle imaging of CNV membranes that appear as hyperreflective bands on OCT. Frequently, the identification of CNV depends on the reflectivity of the adjacent structures and on the CNV localization related to it. OCT is more sensitive than biomicroscopy in identifying retinal edema and small neurosensory and RPE detachments. The OCT relationship with fundus biomicroscopy and fluorescein angiography (FA) in AMD patients is summarized in table 3 [8].

OCT is more reliable than biomicroscopy in assessing the macular thickness and small neurosensory and RPE detachments.
OCT is more reliable than FA in identifying the intraretinal and subretinal fluid, as on FA the fluid in the inner retina can mask the fluid in the outer retina.
OCT is less precise in evaluating the geographic extent of fluid within the macula, as compared to FA.
Due to the cross-sectional imaging, OCT allows the localization of a CNV in relationship with the RPE and the neurosensory retina.
OCT is superior to FA in identifying CNV membranes that are obscured by pooling of dye or by tiny retinal haemorrhages.
Cystoid macular edema is strongly associated with the classic CNV.
OCT is very useful in AMD monitoring and decision-making after treatment: if fluid persists, re-treatment is indicated.

Table 3. Place of OCT in the ophthalmic evaluation of the AMD patients – summary for the clinician

6.2. OCT measurement of macular thickness

In AMD, the most important clinical parameter is the central macular thickness. OCT is the most precise method to measure retinal thickness in vivo. However, OCT measurements cannot be correlated exactly to the histopathologic ones, because OCT signals are directly determined by the optical properties of tissues. Therefore, structures that stain strongly on the histopathological specimens do not necessarily appear as intense OCT signals. It has been demonstrated that there are differences in the retinal thickness measurements between OCT models, possibly explained by the higher axial and transverse resolution of the newer devices. For instance, a comparison was made between Cirrus and Stratus OCT devices in measuring the macular thickness [19]. Firstly, the definition of the retinal boundaries used by the automated segmentation algorithms differs between devices [19]. According to the manufacturer, the Stratus OCT program measures between the nerve fiber layer and the inner boundary of the RPE complex, though it has been reported that Stratus OCT has two outer reference lines: one at the junction between the inner/outer segment of the photoreceptor cells and the other at the inner boundary of the RPE. The Cirrus OCT program measures the retinal thickness between the nerve fiber layer and the outer band of the RPE. In consequence, the Cirrus outer reference band is deeper than the first mentioned Stratus external band and is closer to the second mentioned one. The correlation of thickness measurements between the two devices is modest, as the Cirrus OCT provides greater measurement depth. The practical implications are targeted towards the clinical practice (the patients participating in clinical trials may not interchange between Stratus and Cirrus OCT systems, patients transiting from one practice to another should have the tests done with the same OCT model) and the manufacturer (upgradation of Stratus OCT software). Secondly and more importantly, the TD-OCT calculates the retinal thickness based on 6 radial line scans, whereas SD-OCT uses data of 3D scan with 128-200 scans over the same area [19]. Thus, TD-OCT evaluates a small macular area, whereas SD-OCT images almost the entire macular region.

6.3. OCT imaging of CNV

In neovascular AMD, the retina is invaded by new vessels originating in the choroidal vessels. According to the relationship of these new vessels with the retinal architecture, wet AMD presents in two forms: classic CNV and occult CNV. The histopathological studies proved that in classic CNV the new vessels penetrate Bruch's membrane, the RPE and the neural retina, whereas in occult CNV they are located between the RPE and Bruch's membrane, with subsequent loss of RPE barrier function. In classic CNV the RPE is elevated by exudates, blood and lipids located in the subretinal space and having the origin in the new vessels. The occult CNV can be further divided in two forms: with or without serous pigment epithelial detachment [20] (Table 4). Cystoid macular edema was statistically strongly correlated with the classic form of choroidal neovascularization, whereas the absence of cystoid macular edema was statistically strongly correlated with the occult choroidal neovascular membranes.

CNV type	Location of the new vessels	Clinical findings
Classic	Penetrate Bruch's membrane, RPE, neural retina	RPE elevated by blood, exudates, lipids
Occult	Between Bruch's membrane and RPE	With PED
		Without PED

Table 4. Summary of CNV types – correlation of the histopathological and clinical findings

Occult CNV were described initially on fluorescein angiography (FA) and then on indocyanine green angiography (ICGA) that detected them more accurately, mainly if Scanning Laser Ophthalmoscopy (SLO) was also used. In the recent years, OCT proved its usefulness in defining the features of occult CNV. The main OCT finding that defines occult CNV is the RPE elevation that is separated from the underlying choroidal plane. The cavity formed by the RPE elevation is most frequently fibrovascular and therefore coloured in green, but it can also be serous and then appears optically empty. The RPE elevation is poorly delineated and its extent is variable according to the stage of the lesion. In occult CNV, the RPE elevation can be associated with other OCT signs: modifications of the RPE band (hyperreflectivity, fragmentations, thickening, thinning), subretinal and intraretinal accumulation of fluid, vitreomacular traction syndrome [21].

6.4. OCT in the evaluation of the therapeutical response to photodynamic therapy in wet AMD

OCT helped to better describe the response to treatment in wet AMD. For instance, the response to photodynamic therapy takes place in 5 stages: in the first stage, there is a mild fluid accumulation that corresponds to an acute inflammatory reaction after PDT. Approximately 4 weeks after the first treatment, if there is fluid accumulation, retreatment is suggested. Typically, the fluid accumulates in the subretinal space, causing the detachment of the neurosensory retina. Cystoid macular edema is evident in the penultimate stage, approximately 5 months after PDT and it is associated with important subretinal fibrosis on OCT. In the last stage, there is complete resolution of retinal fluid, concomitant with subretinal fibrosis and retinal atrophy. In conclusion, OCT has a significant impact on the therapeutic approach in AMD: the presence of subretinal fluid proves an active CNV and further therapy is indicated, the presence of fibrosis is associated with cystoid macular edema that has no benefit from therapy as compared to its natural evolution [20].

6.5. OCT imaging of Pigment Epithelial Detachments (PEDs)

In the context of the chorio-retinal diseases, AMD is the condition in which PEDs are the most frequently identified. As hypothesized by Gass, PEDs occur in AMD by two mechanisms: serous exudation from hyperpermeable vessels of the choriocapillaris through an intact Bruch's membrane or neovascular ingrowth with subsequent exudation from the new vessels directly in the subretinal space [22]. Using a TD-OCT device, which was not able to visualize within the PED, Coscas was the first to observe that the presence of a layer of tissue behind the RPE in PEDs is associated with occult CNV. The new devices allow the description of the PEDs content: the dark regions within them are not attributable to the low sensitivity of the imaging technique, but to the hyporeflectivity of the region itself [22]. Before the OCT era, PEDs were assessed manually or automatically according to their areas. However, PEDs can have similar areas but very different volumes, their three-dimensional evaluation being therefore very important. Cirrus SD-OCT system can be used in order to measure the area and volume of PEDs with the help of an algorithm similar to the one reported for the measurement of drusen and that proved to be highly reproducible [23]. The PEDs usually indicate the presence of CNV and are associated with poorer visual outcome. Therefore, their identification carries a prognostic value [22,23].

6.6. OCT imaging of vitreomacular adhesions

Although AMD involves primarily the outer retinal layers, is was suggested by several authors that vitreous may play a role in AMD pathogenesis and/or progression [24]. There is clinical evidence that vitreomacular adhesions may play a role in AMD development. It was proved that the prevalence of PVD was significantly lower in patients with AMD as compared with healthy subjects [25]. In patients with partial PVD, the region of vitreomacular adhesion corresponded to the area of subretinal neovascularization [26]. Also, the incidence of persistent vitreomacular adhesion was significantly higher in eyes with wet AMD as compared to those with dry AMD and controls. Vitreous was also demonstrated to be important in inducing PEDs. If future prospective studies will confirm these findings, it seems appropriate to use OCT in order to assess the vitreomacular relationship in AMD patients. Subsequently, the OCT findings could guide the prevention of wet AMD, by establishing the indication for vitrectomy or pharmacologic vitreolysis [24,25,26].

6.7. Choroidal thickness measurements

Choroid is a very important structure for AMD, because abnormalities at the level of the choroidal circulation seem to be the most significant factor involved in the development of this disease. The use of the newest OCT software enables the measurement of choroidal thickness, but only few studies evaluated it in AMD. So far, it has been proved that the choroidal thickness is variable among patients with AMD. In the group of patients with thicker than normal choroid it is difficult to include them in one of the three following cathegories: a variant of normal, a subset of AMD or a different entity. An overall concluison is that the patients with wet AMD displayed thinner choroids than the ones with dry AMD. These findings postulate that the continuing thinning of the choroid might be a factor indicating the risk of progression towards wet AMD. Therefore, the OCT evaluation of the choroidal thickness could be a valuable tool in identifying the patients at risk to develop the wet form of AMD, thus allowing the early diagnosis and therapy. The thinner than normal choroid induces ischemia at the level of RPE, stimulating the production of VEGF and subsequent proliferation of new vessels. Until now, OCT studies could not establish a correlation between the choroidal thickness and parameters with practical importance: number of intravitreal anti-VEGF injections, duration of the disease, visual acuity [27].

6.8. External retinal cysts

The new OCT imaging techniques allowed to identify the external retinal cysts that differ from the ones in cystoid macular edema and therefore to avoid the useless treatment. They are not perfectly understood yet, but the intravitreal anti-VEGF injections don't seem to influence their evolution. The origin of the external retinal cysts is explained by two theories: inflammatory and mechanical. The inflammatory theory postulates that following photoreceptor and pigment epithelial cells degeneration induced by intravitreal injections of anti-VEGF agents, specific macrophages appear in order to digest the cellular debris. It seems that the external retinal cysts are giant activated macrophages. This theory is sustained by the localization of these cysts in areas of high concentrations of oxidized lipoproteins: in front of the ancient fibro-vascular lesions and of the extended regions of retinal and pigment epithelial atrophy. In accordance with the mechanical theory, the external retinal cysts are rolled photoreceptor cells. During the process of retinal degeneration, the tight junctions between the external segments of the photoreceptor cells disappear and they subsequently form tube-like structures in the external retina. OCT findings exclude the mechanical theory, as the tube-like structures were never identified in AMD, whereas the segmentation OCT techniques proved that the "tubes" correspond to plies of the pigment epithelium and not to rolled photoreceptors. The OCT identification of the external retinal cysts carry an unfavorable prognosis as they are associated with ancient degenerative lesions and with the disappearance of the external retinal layers [3].

6.9. OCT in dry AMD

In dry AMD there is atrophy of the choroid with subsequent degeneration of RPE and involution of the photoreceptor and external retinal layers. However, even if the RPE becomes atrophic, it preserves the barrier function, keeping the macular region dry [20]. The current OCT systems allow the identification of drusen. The small and intermediary size ones appear as discrete elevations of the RPE with variable reflectivity, according to the underlying material. In the large drusen (or so-called drusenoid PEDs) the RPE displays greater, often dome-shaped elevations separated from the Bruch membrane by a hypo or medium reflective material. On OCT images drusen are often accompanied by modifications in the neurosensory retina, translated by the thinning of the outer nuclear layer and disruption at the level of the external limiting membrane and of the inner segment (IS)-outer segment (OS) junctions. These observations are in agreement with the histopathological ones that demonstrated the loss of photoreceptor cells in patients with drusen [28]. Geographic atrophy (GA) appears on OCT as sharply demarcated areas of choroidal hyperreflectivity due to the loss of RPE. If retinal atrophy is associated, thinning or loss of the outer nuclear layer, absence of the external limitting membrane and of the IS-OS junctions are seen. In the areas of GA, islands of preserved retina may be identified, as well as regressing drusenoid materials appearing as hyperreflective plaques at the RPE band. In the GA in the inner nuclear layer may be identified small cystic-like spaces in the absence of any macular edema [28]. The evaluation of GA in terms of size, location and rate of progression is crucial in assessing the visual prognosis of the patients. An important finding that identifies the rapidly progressive cases is the autofluorescence surrounding the GA areas. OCT also revealed in the junctional zones of GA that the outer plexiform layer approaches the Bruch membrane suggesting that photoreceptor loss extends beyond the limits of the lesion. OCT reveals dynamic changes in the junctional zones of GA: pigment migration, variation in drusen height. In conclusion, OCT examination in dry AMD is important in two main directions: it provides insights in the disease pathogenesis and it allows the prediction of visual outcome [28].

6.10. OCT versus angiography in AMD

The advantages of OCT over fluorescein angiography (FA) are represented by: better structural identification of CNV, identification of a CNV masked by the pooling of dye or by thin haemorrhages. On FA, in order to suspect the retinal edema the source of leakage has to be active, whereas on OCT even the minimal edema can be objectivized, no matter if the source of leakage is active or not. Cystoid macular edema in exudative AMD is difficult to be vizualized on FA because of the leakage that obscures the accummulation of fluid in the inner retina. Based on the OCT findings, the prevalence of cystoid macular edema in the cases of subfoveal CNV due to AMD in a retrospective study was estimated to be arround 46%. It has been demonstrated that during all the phases the ICGA substantially underestimated the size of the neovascular complex in comparison to SD-OCT. This could be explained by the high molecular weight and affinity of indocyanine green for the albumin molecules that prevented its even distribution through the entire lesion. Well defined hyperfluorescence during the early phase of FA defining the neovascular complex also underestimated the size of the lesion measured with SD-OCT. On the other hand, despite the SD-OCT capabilities of delivering high resolution images, the components of a fibrovascular complex may represent other subretinal material, particularly of inflammatory origin. Another important observation refers to the extent of leakage during the late phase of FA that did not reach the extension of subretinal or intraretinal fluid objectivized on SD-OCT or even TD-OCT images. It was postulated that minimal fluid on the OCT images might not represent leakage from a newly formed CNV, but failure of liquid resolution by the PRE. Therefore, some authors recommend retreatment by intravitreal anti-VEGF injections only if the presence of fluid on SD-OCT is associated with leakage on FA. However, since SD-OCT is more reliable in detecting extravasated fluid, retreatment based on SD-OCT parameters should be more effective, especially that the pharmacologic therapies act by reducing leakage rather than by an antiproliferative effect [29]. The OCT technology allows new diagnostic criteria for AMD and the decision-making process and AMD monitoring without the need to subject the patient to fluorescein angiography [8]. The ultrahigh-resolution OCT uses a titanium-sapphire laser light source that delivers image resolutions of 3 μm [8]. This is particularly useful in neovascular AMD for the precise evaluation of sub-RPE and sub-foveal choroidal neovascular membranes [8]. On OCT basis, Hee et al. proposed a simple classiffcation scheme of exudative AMD into three categories which does not always correlate with the FA aspects: well-defined CNV, poorly-defined CNV, fibrovascular pigment epithelial detachment. In poorly-defined CNV, the choroidal reflectivity is diffusely increased and is associated with intraretinal or subretinal fluid accummulation that appears hyporeflective. The presence of the fluid or the small disruptions at the level of the RPE or choriocapillaris differentiate the poorly-defined CNV from the RPE atrophy that is translated on OCT as increased choroidal reflectivity as well. The introduction of OCT in the clinical practice was followed by the modification of the classification schemes based on FA. Thus well-defined CNVs or fibrovascular pigment epithelium detachments appear as precisely demarcated boundaries on OCT, whereas on FA sometimes they were classified as occult choroidal neovascular membranes. Poorly-defined CNVs correspond to angiographically occult CNVs in most instances. The emerging conclusion of these practical observations is that OCT provides anatomical details that are not evident on FA. The most important consequence is the optimization at the therapeutic level, as the approaches in angiographically classic and occult CNVs are different [8,29].

7. Stratus OCT in clinical practice

We used the Stratus OCT device (Carl Zeiss Meditech) with the fast macular map scan protocol that consists in 6 radial scans oriented 30 degrees from one another, each having a 2-mm axial depth and 6-mm transverse length. Each image had 10 μm axial and 20 μm transverse resolutions in tissue with a maximum scan velocity of 400 axial scans per second.

Figures 1a and b depict the case of a patient with wet AMD with significantly increased macular thickness (central foveal thickness of 427 μm). Macular edema is provoqued not only by the CNV visible on the cross-sectional images of the retina, but also by an increased vitreo-macular adhesion. The relatively long evolution of the disease is suggested by the modifications in the internal retinal layers, with hyporeflective cysts within their structure. The OCT aspect confirms the theory that the maximal vitreo-macular adhesion is located in front of the subretinal neovascular membrane.

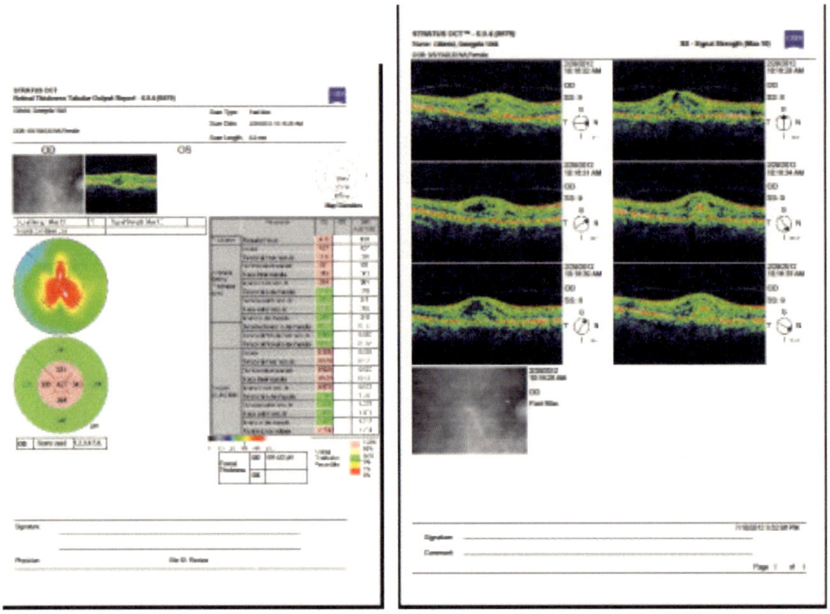

Figure 1. a and b Retinal thickness: increased macular thickness due to CNV but also to vitreo-macular adhesion (courtesy of dr. H. Demea, Review Centre, Cluj-Napoca, Romania)

In figures 2a and b a bilateral AMD case is illustrated. In both eyes the RPE is elevated by a hyperreflective structure (CNV) and the macular thickness is increased. After 2 intravitreal injections with Bevacizumab (Avastin) the RPE elevation and the macular thickness decreased, as shown in figures 3a and b.

Figure 4a shows a macular edema in the left eye of a patient with AMD and figure 4b displays its aspect 20 months after periodic intravitreal injections with Bevacizumab (Avastin). Improvement is obvious, both regarding the central macular thickness and the cross-sectional aspect of the macula. Decision whether to treat or not was based on the OCT aspects, taken on a monthly basis.

The Stratus OCT images in figure 5a and 5b prove an elevation of the RPE in the right eye with moderately increase of central macular thickness (279 μm). One month after intravitreal injection with Bevacizumab (Avastin) the central macular thickness decreased to 246 μm, as shown is figure 6a and 6b.

Figures 7a and 7bare illustrating the Stratus OCT aspects of the left eye of a patient with AMD: there is a marked increase in the central macular thickness (684 μm) and the retinal structure appears disorganized. One year after periodic intravitreal injections with Bevacizumab (Avastin) the central macula appears considerably thinner (380 μm) and the retinal layers much better arranged, as proved in figures 8a and 8b.However, in the internal retinal layers cystic structures appear, suggesting cystoid macular edema. As in case illustrated in figure 4, the decision of treatment was taken exclusively according to the OCT aspects.

http://dx.doi.org/10.5772/53357

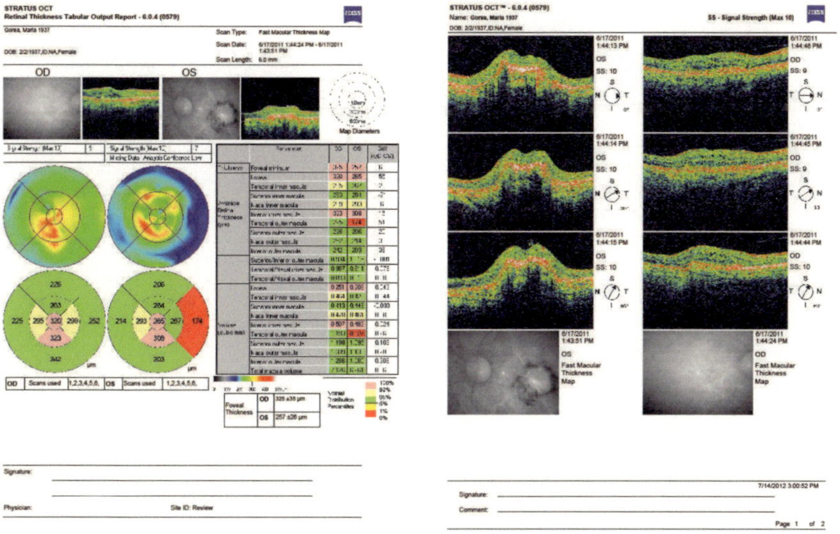

Figure 2. a and b: Patient with bilateral wet AMD before Bevacizumab injections (courtesy of dr. H. Demea, Review Centre, Cluj-Napoca, Romania)

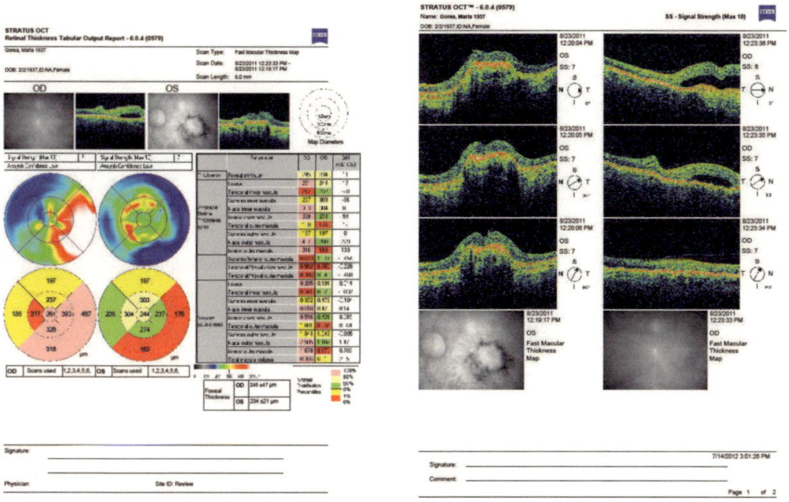

Figure 3. a and b: The case depicted in figure 2, after two intravitreal injections with Bevacizumab (courtesy of dr. H. Demea, Review Centre, Cluj-Napoca, Romania)

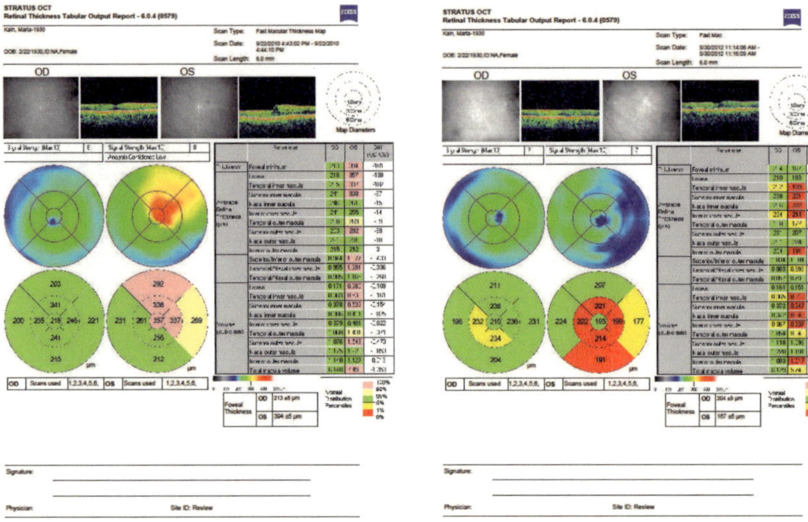

Figure 4. a: Macular edema in AMD (left eye) b: The same patient 20 months after Avastin

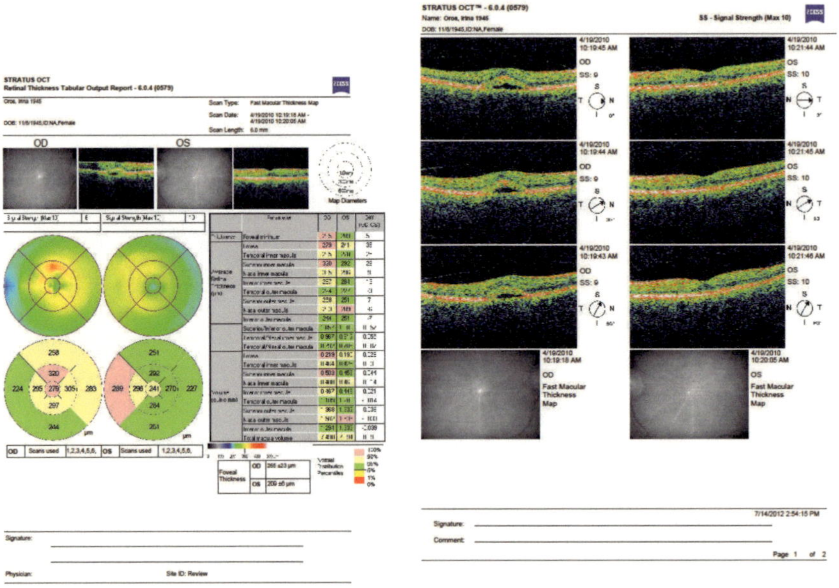

Figure 5. a and b: RPE elevation in AMD patient before Avastin injection (courtesy of dr. H. Demea, Review Centre, Cluj-Napoca, Romania)

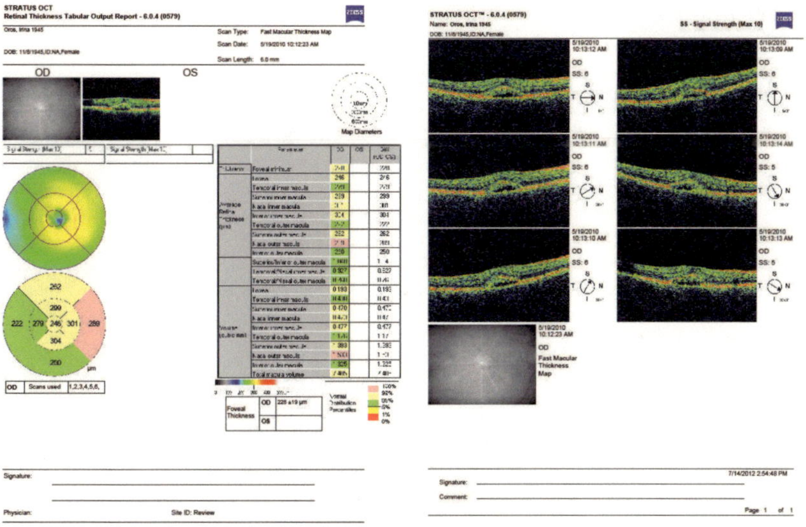

Figure 6. a and b: The case depicted in figure 5, one month after Avastin injection (courtesy of dr. H. Demea, Review Centre, Cluj-Napoca, Romania)

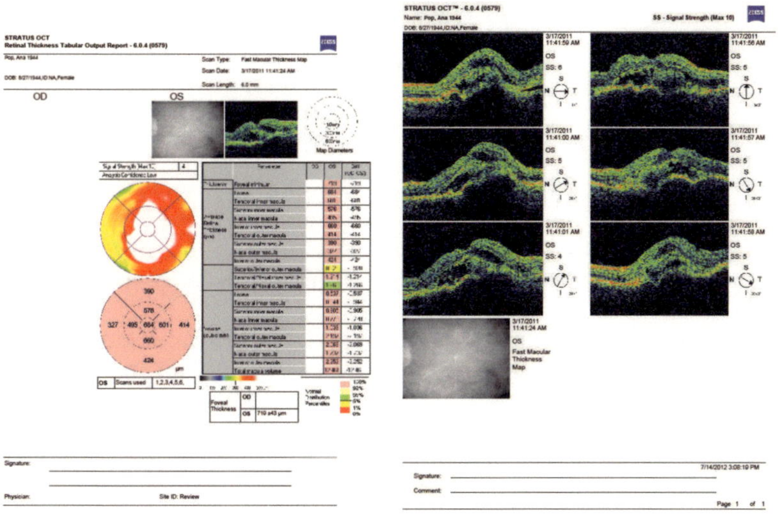

Figure 7. a and b: Advanced case of AMD before Bevacizumab injection

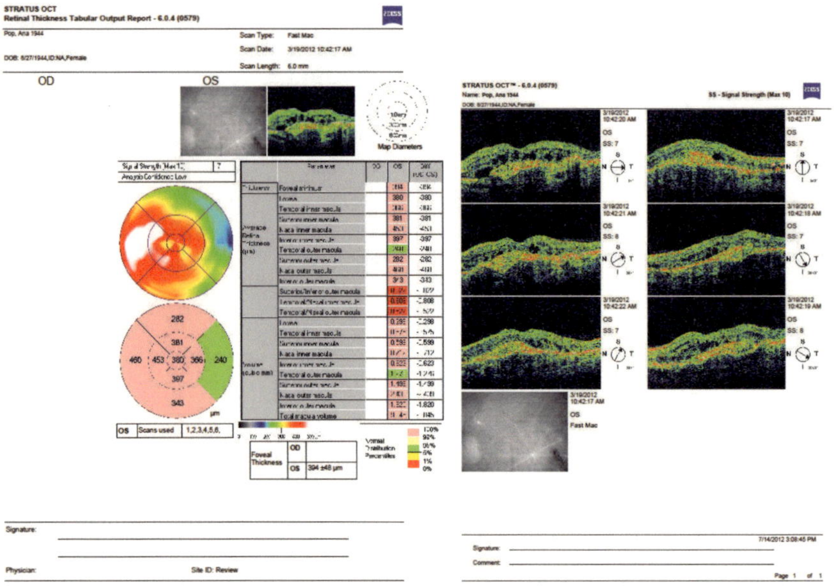

Figure 8. a and b: The same case depicted in figure 7, one year after Avastin injections

8. Cirrus OCT in clinical practice

Average macular thickness is generated automatically with Cirrus-OCT. Each image had a 5 μm axial and 10 μm transverse resolutions in tissue and consisted of either 512 x 128 volume cube or 200 x 200 volume cube with a maximum scan velocity of 27,000 axial scans per second. Cirrus OCT presents high resolution raster scanning capabilities.

Figure 9a presents the HD 5 line raster of a normal retina: the highly reflective retinal layers are red, the layers with intermediate reflectivity are green and the low reflectivity is translated intro blue color. The choriocapillaris under the RPE can also be seen. In figure 9b the macular thickness map and the 512 x 128 volume cube are illustrated.

Figure 10a: irregularities of the RPE band which is elevated by a moderately reflective structure. Behind the RPE band: thick hyperreflective structure. Figure 10b: elevations of the RPE by hyperreflective structures.

Figure 11 illustrates the same patient as in figure 4, with Stratus OCT device. On figure 11a more details are shown, the RPE appears irregular, cysts in the neural retina with a hyporeflective content (fluid) are displayed, not visible on Stratus OCT. Figure 11b presents the macular thickness which is higher than with Stratus OCT. The difference comes from the different boundaries used by the algorihms of the two devices when measuring the macular thickness. The Cirrus OCT program measures the retinal thickness between the nerve fiber layer and the outer band of the RPE. The Stratus OCT program measures between the nerve fiber layer and the inner boundary of the RPE complex, though it has been reported that Stratus OCT has two outer reference lines: one at the junction between the inner/outer segment of the photoreceptor cells and the other at the inner boundary of the RPE. In consequence, the Cirrus outer reference band is deeper than the first mentioned Stratus external band and is closer to the second mentioned one. The correlation of thickness measurements between the two devices is modest, the Cirrus OCT provides greater measurement depth.

Figure 12: irregularities and thinning of the RPE band especially in the right eye, fluid in the retina, increased macular thickness.

Figure 13: RPE band appears thinned and elevated by a moderately reflective tissue: fluid, CNV, increased central macular thickness. 3D macular cube

Figure 14: comparative aspects of the two eyes of the same patient: in the Right Eye the RPE band appears irregular and there is some fluid in the retina.

Figure 15: macular cube 200x200 shows increased central macular thickness, elevations of the RPE band, associated with increased vitreo-macular adhesion revealed by the 3D presentation of the macular cube.

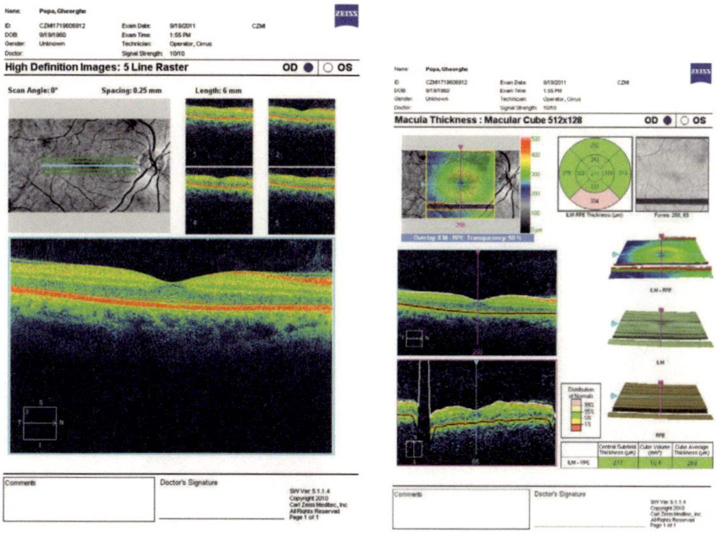

Figure 9. a: 5 line raster of a normal retina b: Normal macular thickness map

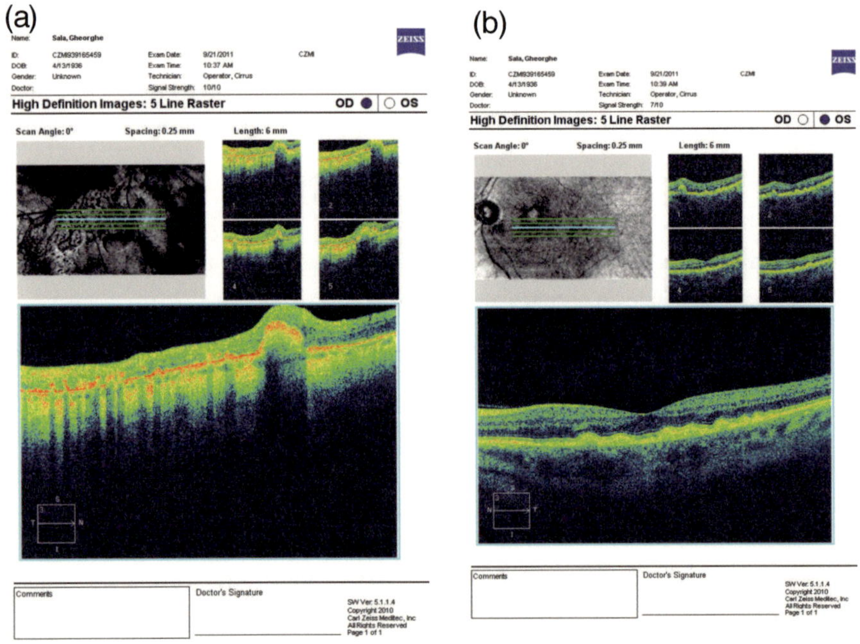

Figure 10. a: Irregularities of the RPE b and b: Elevations of the RPE band

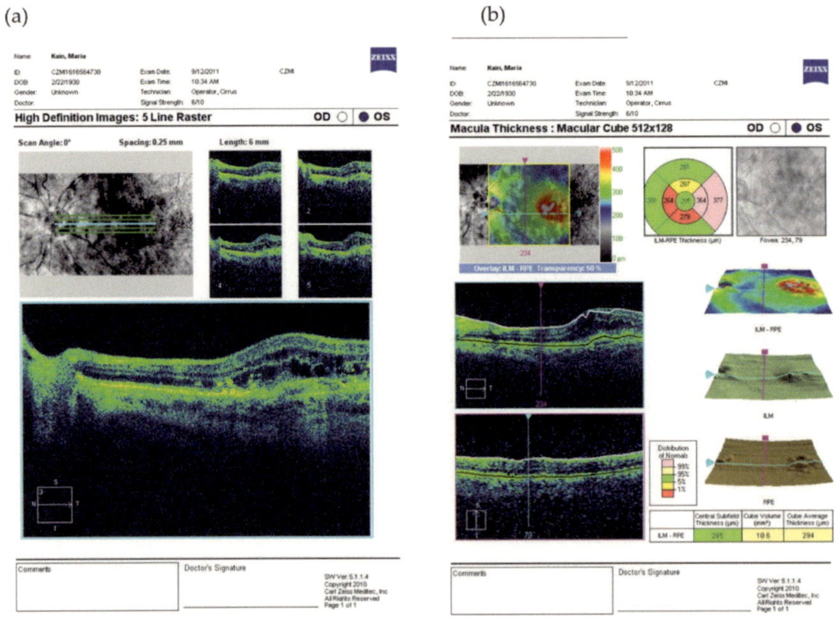

Figure 11. The same patient as in figure 4 a and b

http://dx.doi.org/10.5772/53357

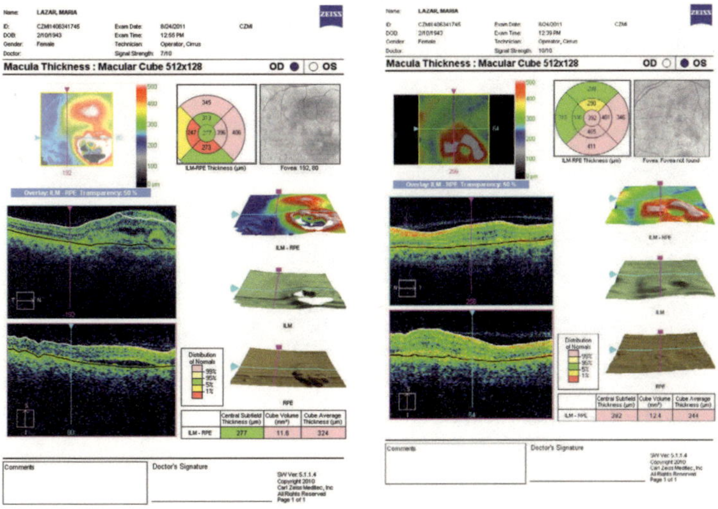

Figure 12. Increased macular thickness, RPE irregularities, fluid in the retina due to AMD

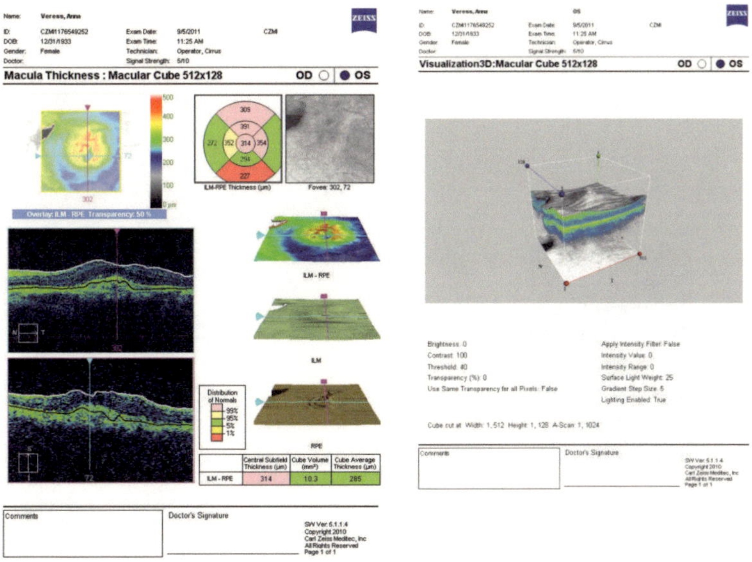

Figure 13. RPE band appears thinned and elevated by a moderately reflective tissue: fluid, CNV, increased central macular thickness. 3D macular cube

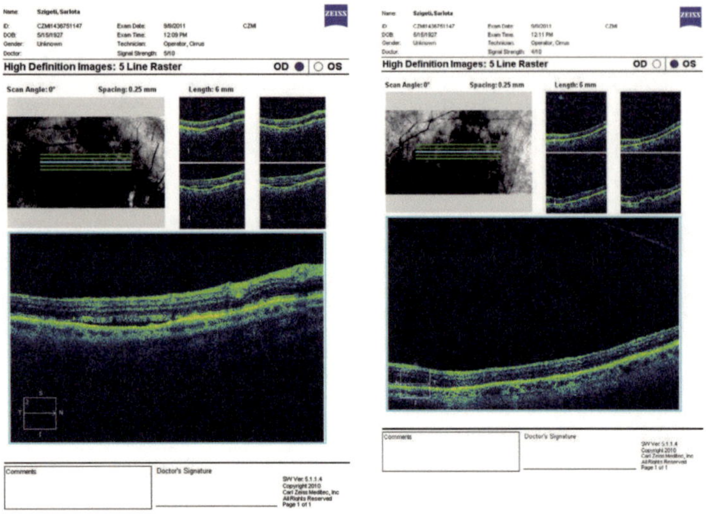

Figure 14. Comparative aspects of the two eyes of the same patient: in the Right Eye the RPE band appears irregular and there is some fluid in the retina.

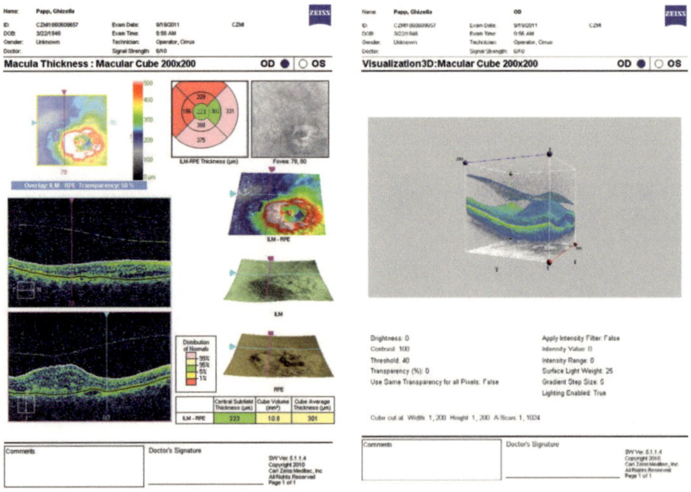

Figure 15. Macular cube 200x200 shows increased central macular thickness, elevations of the RPE band, associated with increased vitreo-macular adhesion revealed by the 3D presentation of the macular cube

9. Future directions

A significant progress for neovascular AMD imaging was the development of FD-OCT technologies. They use a central wavelength of 800-850 nm, a stationary reference arm, a high speed spectrometer and a charged-coupled device (CCD) line-scan camera. The mechanical scanning is not needed in order to detect light echoes simultaneously. As consequence, the aquisition speed increases to 25,000-52,000 A-scan/second. The axial resolution is of 3-7 μm, significantly improving the signal-to-noise ratio and the detection of individual retinal layers and lesions components is possible [16].

9.1. Limits of the current OCT examination techniques

Despite the significant advantages previously mentioned, there are some limitations of SD-OCT: motion and segmentation artifacts, interinstrument comparability [11,12]. Despite the significant progress in retinal imaging offered by the current OCT techniques, TD-OCT and SD-OCT have shortcomings originating in the limitation of resolution, both axial and lateral. The absorbtion of infrared radiation by the anterior segment structures and ocular media limits the image resolution. The axial resolution is limited by the image scattering by the ocular structures (so-called speckle noise) and the lateral resolution limitation is determined by the restricted numerical aperture of the optical system [16].

9.2. Swept source OCT

SS-OCT is another form of FD-OCT that uses a light source with the wavelength of approximately 1,050 nm. A short cavity-swept laser replaces the superluminiscent diode laser. The emission has different frequencies that can be rapidly tuned over a broad bandwidth [11, 28]. A high speed complementary metal oxide semiconductor camera (CMOS) and two parallel photodetectors are used in order to obtain scan rates of 100,000-400,000 A-scan/second, with the axial resolution of 5.3 μm over a 4-mm imaging range.(trebuie modificat) [29]. Advantages: images to the level of individual photoreceptors are obtained, particularly when coupled with adaptive optics. With SS-OCT the so-called fringe washout (signals at the edges of the B-scan) is reduced as compared to SD-OCT; the sensitivity is better with imaging depth; the image range is longer: approximately 7.5 mm, which allows the evaluaiton of the anterior segment without the use of complex imaging techniques that might generate errors [9]; the efficiency of detection is higher; the dual balanced detection can be performed. The above mentioned advantages considerably decrease the patient-induced errors by movements and breathing and permit the better penetration in case of ocular media opacities [30]. Limits: even with best patient cooperation, images are still subject to artifacts. Therefore, various algorithms have been imagined in order to improve the resolution by eliminating these artifacts [30]. The potential application of OCT in the sub-RPE space and choroid is limited by its shallow penetration: approximately 1-3 mm. The degree of choroidal penetration is determined by several factors: the proportion of scattered photons, the absorbtion spectrum of water, the scatter by the ocular media, the absorbtion by melanin [10]. Photon scattering is a phenomenon that influences the image formation in OCT: photons that are singly scattered add to the OCT signal, whereas photons that are scattered multiple times contribute to the background noise [31]. The large amount of water within the eye limits the light wavelengths that can be used [32]. The absorbtion spectrum of water has two regions where the light absorbtion is low: at approximately 950 nm and between 1,000-1,100 nm [30]. The devices with wavelenghts in the range of 1,000-1,100 nm can be used for the enhanced sub-RPE imaging, with ultrahigh-speed image aquisition and axial resolution in the range of 8 μm [10]. This is useful in the managements of sub-RPE space diseases, particularly in AMD.

9.3. Adaptive optics

Adaptive optics correct ocular aberrations during image aquisition, making possible the obtaining of image resolution at the cellular level.

9.4. Enhanced Depth Imaging OCT

The principle of Enhanced depth imaging OCT (EDI-OCT) consists in placing the objective lens of the Spectralis SD-OCT device (Heidelberg Engineering) closer to the eye, with the obtaining of an inverted image, which allows the deeper structures to be placed closer to the zero delay with the subsequent better visualization of the choroid. This principle is combined with the high speed scanning, eye-tracking system, image-averaging technology, reduced noise and greater coverage of the macula. All these improvements lead to the possibility to create high resolution, repeatable and reliable images of the choroid [33].

10. Conclusion

At the present moment, OCT offers the most valuable data on the retinal structure. AMD is the retinal disease that benefited the most from the development of OCT techniques, especially the wet form of this disease. SD-OCT has superior depth resolution as compared to TD-OCT: currently, the axial resolution varies from 3 – 7 μm, depending on the SD-OCT model. OCT is more reliable than biomicroscopy in assessing the macular thickness and small neurosensory and RPE detachments. OCT is more reliable than FA in identifying the intraretinal and subretinal fluid, as on FA the fluid in the inner retina can mask the fluid in the outer retina. OCT is less precise in evaluating the geographic extent of fluid within the macula, as compared to FA. Due to the cross-sectional imaging, OCT allows the localization of a CNV in relationship with the RPE and the neurosensory retina. OCT is superior to FA in identifying CNV membranes that are obscured by pooling of dye or by tiny retinal haemorrhages. Cystoid macular edema is strongly associated with the classic CNV. OCT is very useful in AMD monitoring and decision-making after treatment: if fluid persists, re-treatment is indicated.

http://dx.doi.org/10.5772/53357

Author details

Simona-Delia Ţălu

Address all correspondence to: simonatalu@yahoo.com

Department of Surgical Sciences and Medical Imaging, Ophthalmology, „Iuliu Haţieganu" University of Medicine and Pharmacy, Cluj-Napoca, Romania

References

[1] Lujan B J. Revealing Henle's Fiber Layer Using Spectral-domain OCT. Retin Physician 2011;8(1) 16-17.

[2] Lim LS, Mitchell P, Seddon JM et al. Age-related macular degeneration. Lancet 2012; 379: 1728–38.

[3] El Maftouhi Q, Wolff B, Faysse MM. Kystes rétiniens externes dans la dégénérescence maculaire liée à l'âge exsudative : un nouvel aspect de l'OCT. J Fr d'Ophtalmol. 2010 ;33 : 605-609 doi:10.1016/j.jfo.2010.09.015.

[4] Talu SD, Talu S, Use of OCT Imaging in the Diagnosis and Monitoring of Age Related Macular Degeneration, in Age Related Macular Degeneration.The recent advances in basic research and clinical care, ed. Gui-Shuang Ying, Rijeka, Intech, 2012.

[5] Huang D, Swanson EA, Lin CP et al. Optical coherence tomography. Science 1991;22 1178-1181.

[6] Hee MR, Puliafito CA, Wong C et al. Quantitative assessment of macular edema with optical coherence tomography. Arch Ophthalmol. 1995;113 1019 – 1029.

[7] Ghazi N, Kirk T, Allam S et al. Quantification of Error in Optical CoherenceTomography Central Macular Thickness Measurement in Wet Age-related Macular Degeneration. Am J Ophthalmol 2009;148:90–96 doi:10.1016/j.ajo.2009.02.017

[8] F. G.Holz R. F. Spaide. Essentials in ophthalmology. Medical Retina, Berlin Heidelberg, 2005

[9] Costa RA, Skaf M, Melo LA Jr et al. Retinal assessment using optical coherence tomography. Prog Retin Eye Res. 2006;25 325-353.

[10] Keane PA, Ruiz-Garcia H, Sadda SR. Clinical applications of long-wavelength (1,000-nm) optical coherence tomography. Ophthalmic Surg Lasers Imaging 2011;42 S67-S74.

[11] Potsaid B, Baumann B, Huang D et al. Ultrahigh speed 1050nm speedswept source/ Fourier domain OCT retinal and anterior segment imaging at 100,000 to 400,000 axial scans per second. Opt Express. 2010;18 20029-20048

[12] Sull AC, Vuong LN, Price LL et al. Comparison of spectral/Fourier domain optical coherence tomography instruments for assessment of of normal macular thickness. Retina 2010;30 235-245.

[13] Menke M, Lala C, Framme C, Wolf S. The Ever-Evolving Role of Imaging in DME Management. Retin Physician 2012;9(4) 24-32.

[14] Lumbroso B, Rippoli M. Guide to Interpreting Spectral Domain Optical Coherence Tomography. James Allyn, Inc.; Dublin, CA; 2010

[15] Kiernan DF, Mieler WF, Hariprasad SM. Spectral-Domain Optical Coherence Tomography: A Comparison of Modern High-Resolution Retinal Imaging Systems Am J Ophthalmol 2010;149:18–31 doi:10.1016/j.ajo.2009.08.037

[16] Wojkowski M, Kaluzny B, ZawadziRJ. New directions in ophthalmic optical coherence tomography. Optom Vis Sci 2012 Mar 22 (Epub ahead of print).

[17] Murakami T, Nishijima K, Akagi T et al. Optical coherence tomographic reflectivity of photoreceptors beneath cystoid spaces in diabetic macular edema. Invest Ophthalmol Vis Sci 2012 Feb 8 (epub ahead of print)

[18] Salam A, Framme C, Wolf S. How SD-OCT is changing our view of DME. Retin Physician 2010;7(8) 41-46.

[19] Kiernan DF, Hariprasad HM, Chin EK et al. Prospective Comparison of Cirrus and Stratus Optical Coherence Tomography for Quantifying Retinal Thickness. Am J Ophthalmol. 2009;147 267-275 doi:10.1016/j.ajo.2008.08.018

[20] Philip L. Penfold, Jan M. Provis. Macular Degeneration. Springer, Berlin Heidelberg, 2005.

[21] Sulzbacher F, Kiss C, Munk M et al. Diagnostic Evaluation of Type 2 (Classic) Choroidal Neovascularization: Optical Coherence Tomography, Indocyanine Green Angiography, and Fluorescein Angiography. Am J Ophthalmol. 2011;152:799–806 doi: 10.1016/j.ajo.2011.04.011

[22] Spaide RF. Enhanced Depth Imaging Optical Coherence Tomography of Retinal Pigment Epithelial Detachment in Age-related Macular Degeneration. Am J Ophthalmol 2009;147:644–652 doi:10.1016/j.ajo.2008.10.005

[23] Penha FM, Rosenfeld PJ, Gregori G et al. Quantitative Imaging of Retinal Pigment Epithelial Detachments Using Spectral-Domain Optical Coherence Tomography. Am J Ophthalmol 2012;153:515–523 doi:10.1016/j.ajo.2011.08.031

[24] Mojana F, Cheng L, Bartsch DUG et al. The Role of Abnormal Vitreomacular Adhesion in Age-related Macular Degeneration: Spectral Optical Coherence Tomography

and Surgical Results. Am J Ophthalmol. 2008;146: 218-227 doi:10.1016/j.ajo.2008.04.027

[25] Lee SJ, Lee CS, Koh HJ. Posterior Vitreomacular Adhesion and Risk of Exudative Age-related Macular Degeneration: Paired Eye Study. Am J Ophthalmol. 2009; 147: 621-626, doi:10.1016/j.ajo.2008.10.003

[26] Krebs I, Brannath W, Glittenberg C et al. Posterior Vitreomacular Adhesion: A Potential Risk Factor for Exudative Age-related Macular Degeneration? Am J OPhthalmol. 2007; 144: 741-746 doi:10.1016/j.ajo.2007.07.024

[27] Manjunath V, Goren J, Fujimoto FJ et al. Analysis of Choroidal Thickness in Age-Related Macular Degeneration Using Spectral-Domain Optical Coherence Tomography. Am J Ophthalmol 2011;152: 663–668 doi:10.1016/j.ajo.2011.03.008

[28] Keane PA. Sadda SR. Predicting visual outcomes for macular disease using optical coherence tomography. Saudi Journal of Ophthalmology. 2011;25 145-158 doi: 10.1016/j.sjopt.2011.01.003

[29] Regatieri CV, Branchini L, Duker JS. The role of spectral-domain OCT in the diagnosis and management of neovascular age-related macular degeneration. Ophthalmic Sur Lasers Imaging. 2011 42 S56-S66.

[30] Raiji V, Walsh A, Sadda S. Future Directions in Retinal Optical Coherence Tomography. Retin Physician 2012;9(4) 33-37.

[31] Sharma U, Chang EW, Yun SH. Long-wavelength optical coherence tomography at 1.7 microm for enhanced imaging depth. Opt Express. 2008; 16 19712-19723.

[32] Unterhuber A, Povazay B, Hermann B, Sattmann H, Chavez-Pirson A, Drexler W. In vivo retinal optical coherence tomography at 1040 nm; enhanced penetration into the choroid. Opt Express. 2005; 13 3252-3258.

[33] Spaide RF, Koisumi H, Posonni MC. Enhanced depth imaging spectral-domain optical coherence tomography. Am J Ophthalmol. 2008; 146 496-500.

Section 3

New Trend in the Management of AMD

Chapter 5

Anti VEGF Agents for Age Related Macular Degeneration

Shani Golan, Michaella Goldstein and Anat Loewenstein

Additional information is available at the end of the chapter

http://dx.doi.org/10.5772/54198

1. Introduction

The adult retina is a neural tissue with high metabolism and the highest oxygen consumption per unit weight of all human tissues. Therefore, the choroid, the most vascular layer of the eye also nourishing the retina, has one of the highest blood-flow rates in the body, 800 – 1000 mL/100 g tissue/min [1]. In healthy adults this delicate ocular vascular system is maintained and controlled by the balance between the angiogenic factors and angiogenic inhibitors [2].

Age-related macular degeneration (AMD) is the result of complex interactions between lipofuscinogenesis, drusenogenesis, and inflammation which can lead to choroidal neovascularization(CNV)[3]. An imbalance between the proangiogenic vascular endothelial growth factor (VEGF) and the antiangiogenic pigment epithelium-derived factor (PEDF)[3-4], plays a major role in the pathogenesis of the disease.

Inhibitors of VEGF represent a relatively new treatment for CNV. These agents include the Macugen (aptamer) which was almost completely abandoned with the introduction of the efficient FDA approved Ranibizumab (Lucentis; Genentech, Inc, South San Francisco, CA), in addition to others such as the Bevacizumab (Avastin; Genentech, Inc), and the new FDA approved drug Eylea(VEGF Trap Eye Regeneron, Tarrytown, NY, USA).

2. Vascular endothelial growth factors

Vascular endothelial growth factor (VEGF) plays a key role in ocular angiogenesis and vascular permeability. Several VEGF family members have been discovered (VEGF-A, B, C, D and PIGF). These isoforms of VEGF have different effects in ocular pathologies and may differ in their neuroprotective abilities [5, 6]. RPE and Müller cells are the major sources of VEGF and they exert their effects through multiple receptors that are mostly expressed on endothelial cells and are also found on monocytes and macrophages [7].

VEGF-A, has been most strongly associated with angiogenesis and thus consists the target of most anti-VEGF treatments [8, 9]. VEGF-A signals through two receptor tyrosine kinases, VEGFR1 and VEGFR2, and is induced by hypoxia, unlike other VEGF isoforms [7, 10].

Alternative exon splicing of the human VEGF-A gene results in at least four major biologically active isoforms, containing 121, 165, 189, and 208 aminoacids (five more are VEGFA-145, VEGFA-162, VEGFA-165b, VEGFA-183, and VEGFA-206) [11].

Different VEGF-A isoforms may have different functions in ocular diseases.

VEGF 121 appears to be essential for normal retinal vascular function [12-13], and VEGFA-165 is the predominant isoform in the human eye. It isa heparin-binding, homodimeric, 45-kDa glycoprotein that is predominantly secreted, although a substantial fraction is bound to the cell surface and to the extracellular matrix[13-14].It appears to be the isoform responsible for pathological ocular neovascularization.

Both isoforms are found in CNV tissue excised from patients with AMD.

In autopsy studies, VEGF levels were found to be elevated in the retinal pigment epithelium (RPE) and choroidal blood vessels within the macular area of eyes with AMD [15].

In summary VEGF-A acts through various pathways which result in promoting pathologic neovascularization:

- It stimulates angiogenesis by being a potent endothelial cell mitogen [10-11].
- It sustains endothelial survival by inhibiting apoptosis [10-12].
- VEGF is a chemo-attractant for endothelial cell precursors, promoting their differentiation [12-13].
- It is a powerful agonist of vascular permeability which is particularly important in CNV. Increased vascular permeability in response to VEGF may be due to formation of fenestrations in microvascular endothelium [12-14].
- Leukocytes may amplify the effects of VEGF via their own secretion of VEGF. Furthermore, VEGF's pro-inflammatory activity, predominantly through the 164 isoform, contributes to pathological ocular neovascularization [14]. It is therefore a crucial target in combating neovascular and ischemic eye diseases such as: choroidal neovascularization, macular edema secondary to diabetic retinopathy (DME) or retinal vein occlusion and retinal neovascularisation that may develop in retinal vein occlusion (RVO) or diabetic retinopathy (DR).

Several anti-VEGF drugs have been studied and have been shown to be effective. However, effective, long-term drug-delivery remains a challenge. Two multi-center, randomized controlled trials comparing the two most commonly drugs available were published recently. A summary of the available drugs (table 1), their mechanism of action and results from large multicenter trials evaluating their efficacy and safety is presented below.

3. Anti VEGF drugs

3.1. Pegaptanib sodium (Macugen) – OSI/Eyetech

This intravitreal RNA aptamer drug was the first anti-VEGF drug approved by the FDA in 2004 for use in neovascular AMD (nvAMD). It targets VEGFA-$_{165}$[11]Its efficacy and safety were evaluated in the large VISION trial [16, 17].

Patients with different types of sub foveal CNV secondary to AMD were randomized into four groups. Three groups received an intravitreal injection of pegaptanib sodium at a dose of 0.3mg, 1.0mg, 3.0mg to one eye respectively. The injection was given every 6 weeks for a period of 48 weeks in total. The forth group was the control group and subjects in this group received a sham injection every 6 weeks. Primary outcome was mean change in visual acuity from baseline.

Results from a combined analysis showed that for all three doses of pegaptanib ($P<0.001$ for the comparison of 0.3 mg with sham injection; $P<0.001$ for the comparison of 1.0 mg with sham injection; and $P=0.03$ for the comparison of 3.0 mg with sham injection) there was a significant difference between the patients receiving treatment and those receiving a sham injection. In the group dosed with pegaptanib 0.3 mg, 70 percent of patients lost fewer than 15 letters of visual acuity (VA), as compared with 55 percent among the controls ($P<0.001$). The risk of severe loss of VA (loss of 30 letters or more) was reduced from 22 percent in the sham-injection group to 10 percent in the group receiving 0.3 mg of pegaptanib ($P<0.001$). More patients receiving pegaptanib (0.3 mg), as compared with sham injection, maintained their VA or gained acuity (33 % vs. 23%; $P=0.003$). As early as six weeks after beginning therapy with the study drug, and at all subsequent points, the mean visual acuity among patients receiving 0.3 mg of pegaptanib was better than in those receiving sham injections ($P<0.002$). During the second year, patients initially assigned to pegaptanib were re-randomized (1:1) to continue or discontinue therapy for 48 additional weeks (8 injections). Those initially assigned to sham were re-randomized to continue sham, discontinue sham, or receive 1 of 3 pegaptanib doses. The proportion of patients who lost more than 15 letters or more in vision between week 52 to week 96 was double (14 *vs* 7%), if treatment was discontinued compared to those who continued to receive pegaptanib injections. This suggests that there is a more favorable outcome when continuing treatment for at least two years [18].The Pegaptanib was found safe and there was no significant difference in serious systemic adverse events or severe ocular inflammation, cataract or glaucoma between the pegaptanib treated groups and the sham treated groups [16, 17].

The VA results of the VISION study are clearly inferior to those of the MARINA and ANCHOR studies evaluating the efficacy of intravitreal ranibizumab for nvAMD (detailed later). However, VA efficacy is only one of the clinical considerations that must be taken into account. The safety profile of the drug is not less important. The Macugen was proven to be safe in the VISION study as well as in the smaller study by N. Feucht et al. [19]; in both studies no relevant systemic or ocular adverse effects were noted. Cardiovascular incidents and overall mortality in the Pegaptanib sodium group were comparable to those of the sham injection group.

Thus, we can conclude that stable vision can be achieved with repeated injections as frequent as every 6 weeks with pegaptanib. This treatment may still be taken into consideration especially in subjects suffering from cardiovascular diseases.

3.2. Ranibizumab (Lucentis) - Genentech

Ranibizumab is a small 48kDa recombinant humanized monoclonal antibody fragment. Its small molecular weight enables it to penetrate the inner limiting membrane and reach the subretinal space when injected intravitreally [5,8-9]. It binds all biologically active isotypes of VEGF with high affinity. The half-life of ranibizumab is 2 – 4 days [5, 8], resulting in a rapid systemic clearance and good systemic safety profile.

FDA has approved the use of ranibizumab for treatment of all angiographic subtypes of subfoveal CNV due to AMD. The phase III MARINA trial evaluated the efficacy and safety of ranibizumab for the treatment of minimally classic or occult with no classic CNV associated with AMD. This 2-year, prospective randomized, double-masked, sham-controlled trial enrolled 716 patients. Patients were randomized in a 1 : 1 : 1 ratio to receive intravitreal ranibizumab at a dose of either 0.3 mg or 0.5mg or sham injection monthly in one eye for 2 years [9]. The primary outcome was the proportion of patients losing fewer than 15 letters from baseline visual acuity at 12 months.

At 24 months, 92% of patients who received 0.3 mg of ranibizumab and 90% of patients who received 0.5 mg ranibizumab lost fewer than 15 letters, compared with 52.9% in the sham group. The proportion of patients who gained at least 15 letters on the Early Treatment of Diabetic Retinopathy Study (ETDRS) chart from baseline to 24 months was 33.3% in the 0.5mg group, 26.1% in the 0.3mggroup, and 3.8% in the sham group. The mean change in ETDRS VA from baseline to 24 months was a gain of 6.6 letters in the 0.5mg group, a gain of 5.4 letters in the 0.3mg group, and a loss of 14.9 letters in the sham-injection group [9].

The ANCHOR study evaluated the efficacy of Ranibizumab for treatment of Predominantly Classic sub foveal CNV due to AMD. The ANCHOR trial was a multicenter, randomized double-blind trial that enrolled 423 patients to compare the efficacy and safety of ranibizumab vs PDT with verteporfin[20]. Patients were assigned randomly to receive either 0.3 or 0.5mg of ranibizumab plus sham verteporfin, or sham intravitreal injection plus active verteporfin therapy. Ranibizumab or sham intravitreal injections were given monthly, and the verteporfin or sham was administered on day 0 and then as needed at months 3,6, 9, and 12.

At 12 months, 94.3% of patients in the 0.3mg group and96.4% in the 0.5mg group lost fewer than 15 letters from baseline compared with 64.3% in the verteporfin group. The proportion of patients who gained at least 15 letters from baseline to 12 months was

40.3% in the 0.5mg group, 35.7%in the 0.3mg group, and 5.6% in the verteporfin group. The mean change in VA from baseline to 12months was a gain of 8.5 letters in the 0.3mg group, a gain of11.3 letters in the 0.5mg group, and a loss of 9.5 letters in the verteporfin group [20]. Rates of serious ocular or systemic adverse events were low in both the MARIMA and the ANCHOR trials[20].

Both studies showed no difference in the percentage of patients losing 15 letters in vision between the 0.3 and 0.5mg. However, the 0.5 mg was statistically significant superior to the 0.3 mg in achieving 15 letters or more in vision. This difference in favor of the 0.5 mg led to its approval by the FDA, and the routine use of 0.5 mg ranibizumab.

The PIER study [21] evaluated the efficacy of 3 consecutive monthly injections of ranibizumab followed by fixed re-treatments only every 3 months. Mean changes from baseline VA at 12 months were -16.3, -1.6, and -0.2 letters loss for the sham, 0.3 mg, and 0.5 mg groups, respectively (P < or =.0001, each ranibizumab dose vs sham). Ranibizumab reduced the growth and leakage from the CNV. However, the treatment effect achieved following the first 3 consecutive injections declined in the ranibizumab groups during quarterly dosing (e.g., at three months the mean changes from baseline VA was a gain of 2.9 and 4.3 letters for the 0.3 mg and 0.5 mg doses, respectively). Results of subgroups analyses of mean change from baseline VA at 12 months by baseline age, VA, and lesion characteristics were consistent with the overall results. Overall, in this study, the proportion of gainers of more than three lines was significantly lower than in MARINA or in ANCHOR trials, and this is due to the fact that following the first 3 consecutive injections patients were shifted to a significant less frequent dosing of quarterly injections instead of monthly.

The EXCITE study evaluated the efficacy and safety of monthly versus quarterly ranibizumab treatment in nvAMD [22]. Patients were randomized (1:1:1) to 0.3 mg quarterly, 0.5 mg quarterly, or 0.3 mg monthly doses of ranibizumab. Treatment comprised of a loading phase (3 consecutive monthly injections) followed by a 9-month maintenance phase (either monthly or quarterly injection).In contrast to the PIER study in which patients were examined and injected only every 3 months following the first 3 consecutive monthly injections, in the EXCITE study, patients were followed monthly, but in the 2 quarterly groups they could receive an injection only every 3 months. BCVA increased from baseline to month 12 by 4.9, 3.8, and 8.3 letters in the 0.3 mg quarterly (104 patients), 0.5 mg quarterly (88 patients), and 0.3 mg monthly (101 patients) dosing groups, respectively. The noninferiority of a quarterly regimen was not achieved with reference to 5.0 letters, meaning dosing with ranibizumab only every 3 months is inferior than dosing every month, and results in a significant less favorable final visual outcome. The safety profile was similar to that reported in prior ranibizumab studies.

Following the results of the PIER and EXCITE study it can be concluded that monthly injections is definitely superior to quarterly injections, and that the quarterly regimen should not be applied.

3.3. Bevacizumab (Avastin) - Genentech

This drug is a full-length recombinant humanized monoclonal antibody (149kDa).It binds to all VEGF-A isoforms. whereas Ranibizumab has only one binding site to VEGF, bevacizumab has two. Bevacizumab in addition has a longer acting effect *in-vitro*; however, it may penetrate less effectively the retina [23-26]. Its half life time in the vitreous is approximately 8-10 days [24-25].

It was first approved by the FDA for metastatic colorectal cancer and is used off-label in ocular disease. Although systemic administration of bevacizumab was shown to be associated with increased systemic cardiovascular adverse events, these appear to be rare following intravitreal administration [8, 24].

Many ophthalmologists until recently offered intravitreal bevacizumab to nvAMD patients based on multiple forms of evidence: results from several retrospective case series,[27-30] extrapolation from the outcomes reported in the MARINA and ANCHOR studies, the structural similarity between ranibizumab and bevacizumab, and mostly the clinical experience of rapid resolution of morphological abnormalities on optical coherence tomography (OCT) and fluorescein leakage from CNV after treatment with bevacizumab.

However, treatment with bevacizumab can nowdays be based on the 2-year results of the Comparison of Age-Related Macular Degeneration Treatment Trial (CATT) and one year results of IVAN study (Inhibit VEGF in Age-related choroidal Neovascularisation)which compared the efficacy of bevacizumab and ranibizumab for nvAMD and will be discussed in detail later in this chapter.

3.4. Aflibercept (VEGF trap)

VEGF Trap-Eye (EYLEA; Regeneron, Tarrytown, NY, USA) (VTE) is a soluble fusion protein consisting of 2 extracellular cytokine receptor domains and a human Fc region of immunoglobulin G (IgG). This110kDa soluble receptor binds with high affinity to all VEGFA isoforms and VEGF B, and not to VEGF-C and D [5]. The binding affinity of VEGF Trap to VEGF is 10 times higher than bevacizumab. The 2mg dose of VTE at 83days has been proven to have a similar biologic activity to ranibizumab at 30 days [5, 31]. The CLEAR-IT is a phase II trial, which was recently published and evaluated anatomic outcomes and VA, injection frequency, and safety. The study consisted of 2 phases; the first was a 12-week fixed dosing period followed by an as-needed (PRN) treatment phase to week 52 with VEGF Trap-Eye for nvAMD [31]. Patients were randomly assigned to 1 of 5 intravitreal VEGF Trap-Eye treatment groups: 0.5 mg or 2 mg every 4 weeks or 0.5, 2, or 4 mg every 12 weeks during the fixed-dosing period (weeks 1-12). From weeks 16 to 52, patients were evaluated monthly and were retreated PRN with their assigned dose (0.5, 2, or 4 mg). The decrease in CR/LT (central retinal/lesion thickness) at week 12 versus baseline remained significant at weeks 12 to 52 (-130 μm from baseline at week 52) and CNV size regressed from baseline by 2.21 mm^2at 48 weeks. After achieving a significant improvement in BCVA during the 12-week- fixed-dosing phase for all groups combined, PRN dosing for 40 weeks maintained the improvement in BCVA to 52 weeks (5.3-letter gain; P<0.0001). The robust improvement and consistent maintenance of VA mainly occurred in patients initially dosed with 2 mg every 4 weeks for 12 weeks, demonstrating a gain of 9 letters at 52 weeks. Overall, a mean of 2 injections was administered after the 12-week fixed-dosing phase, and the mean time to first reinjection was 129 days; 19% of patients received no injections and 45% received 1 or 2 injections. Treatment with VEGF Trap-Eye was generally safe and well tolerated, with few ocular or systemic adverse events. They concluded that PRN dosing with VEGF Trap-Eye at weeks 16-52 maintained the significant anatomic and visual improvements established during the 12-week fixed-dosing phase with a low need for re-injections. Repeated dosing with VEGF Trap-Eye was well tolerated over 52 weeks of treatment.

VIEW1 was a phase III non-inferiority trial conducted in North America that randomized 1217 patients to VTE 0.5 mg monthly dosing (0.5q4wk), VTE 2 mg monthly (2q4wk),VTE 2 mg every two months following 3 initial monthly doses (2q8wk), or ranibizumab 0.5mg monthly (Rq4wk). The primary endpoint was the proportion of patients who lost fewer than 15 ETDRS letters from baseline to week 52 [32].

Secondary endpoints included mean change in BCVA at week 52. The percentage of participants in the Rq4wk, 0.5q4wk, 2q4wk, and 2q8wk treatment arms who gained at least 15 letters in vision were: 31%,25%, 38%, and 31%, respectively.

The proportions of patients maintaining vision at 52 weeks were 94.4%, 95.9%, 95.1%, and 95.1% for Rq4wk, 0.5q4wk, 2q4wk, and 2q8wk, respectively. All VTE groups were noninferior to ranibizumab. Mean improvement from baseline to week 52 in ETDRS letter score was 8.1, 6.9, 10.9, and 7.9 letters for Rq4wk, 0.5q4wk, 2q4wk, and 2q8wk, respectively.

There was a small significant difference in visual improvement at 52 weeks, between the 2q4wk and the Rq4weeks in favor of the 2q4weeks, however this was not found in the parallel VIEW 2 trial that will be discussed later. Differences between other VTE groups and Rq4wk were nonsignificant. The difference in the mean reduction in central retinal thickness was not significant among the groups. The incidence of adverse events was similar across all treatments, with no increase in blood pressure noted.

Overall, dosing monthly or every two months with VTE was non-inferior to monthly ranibizumab and was well tolerated [32]. The VIEW2 study was a parallel study to VIEW 1 that enrolled 1240 patients from Europe, Latin America, Asia, and Australia and yielded similar results [33]. However, minor differences exist. In the VIEW 2 study there was no statistically significant difference between all treatment arms in ETDRS letter score at week 52, and unlike VIEW1 the 2q4wk group was not superior to Lucentis.

The VIEW 1 and VIEW 2 results demonstrated non-inferior efficacy of VTE 2mg dosed at a fixed regimen every 8 weeks compared to ranibizumab 0.5mg dosed every 4 weeks. The EYLEA was approved by the FDA for injection every 8 weeks for nvAMD, and therefore may lower the injection burden on the patient as well as the medical system.

4. Different regimens for Bevacizumab and Ranibizumab

4.1. Ranibizumab: As-needed regimen

Numerous studies evaluated the effect of PRN intravitreal ranibizumab for the treatment of nvAMD.

The Prospective OCT Imaging of Patients with nvAMD Treated with Intraocular Ranibizumab (PrONTO) study was the first open-label, prospective, uncontrolled study to investigate a variable-dosing of intravitreal ranibizumab over two years [34]. Thirty-seven patients received 3 consecutive monthly injections of 0.5 mg ranibizumab and were then followed monthly and re-treated if there was an increase in OCT central retinal thickness (CRT) of at least 100 microns or a loss of BCVA of 5 letters or more. During the second year, the retreatment criteria were amended to include re-treatment if any qualitative increase in the amount of fluid was detectedon OCT. At 24 months (end of 2 years study), mean VA improved by 11letters with an average of 9.9 injections In the PrONTO study therefore we can conclude that VA outcomes were nearly comparable with those reported in the MARINA and ANCHOR, but these results were achieved with less than half number of intravitreal injections given in the MARINA and ANCHOR[34].

The SUSTAIN trial was a phase III multicenter open-label single arm study that assessed the safety and efficacy of ranibizumab in patients with sub foveal CNV secondary to AMD using a dosing regimen individualized to patient characteristics. 513 patients who were either ranibizumab treatment –naïve (69 patients) or had completed treatment with ranibizumab or verteporfin PDT in the ANCHOR trial participated in this study [35].

Patients received three consecutive monthly injections of ranibizumab 0.3mg (or 0.5mg for the ANCHOR patients) (the "loading phase"), followed by monthly monitoring visits. Further treatment was administered if VA decreased by >5 letters or if CRT increased by >100 μm. Compared with baseline, mean VA at month 12 increased by approximately 7 letters. VA reached a maximum level after the first 3 monthly injections, decreased slightly when shifting to PRN during the next 2 to 3 months and was then sustained throughout the treatment period. Over 12 months, the mean standard deviation (SD) number of ranibizumab injections received by the 69 ranibizumab naıve patients was 5.3 (±2.2), including the three "loading" injections. This study demonstrated that flexible, guided dosing with fewer injections and monthly monitoring can be efficient and result in good visual outcome in at least some patients [35].

The SAILOR (Safety Assessment of IntravitrealLucentis for age-related macular degeneration) study, a Phase IIIb study of Lucentis for patients with all subtypes of new or recurrent active sub fovealCNV due to AMD, was a twelve-month randomized (cohort 1) or open-label (cohort 2) multicenter clinical trial [36]. 4300 subjects were recruited. Cohort 1 subjects were randomized 1:1 to receive 0.3 mg (n = 1169) or 0.5 mg (n = 1209) intravitreal ranibizumab for 3 monthly loading doses, followed by monthly visits. Cohort 2 subjects received 1 single open-label 0.5 mg intravitreal ranibizumab, and than continue the monthly follow up visits. Those groups were stratified by AMD treatment history (treatment-naïve vs. previously treated). Cohort 1 subjects were retreated on the basis of OCT or BCVA criteria. Cohort 2 subjects (n = 1922) received an initial single intravitreal dose of 0.5 mg ranibizumab and were retreated at physician discretion. Safety was evaluated at all visits. It concluded that Intravitreal ranibizumab was safe and well tolerated in a large population of subjects with neovascular AMD. Ranibizumab had a beneficial effect on VA but quarterly visits were insufficient to monitor and capture disease progression [36] If a fixed regimen of monthly injections is not applied, than monthly visits are recommended and injectios performed as needed usually guided by visual acuity and OCT findings.

The HORIZON study was an open-label multicenter extension study that included 853 patients (600 had been previously treated with ranibizumab initially, 184 had crossed over to treatment with ranibizumab, and 69 had not been treated with ranibizumab) who had completed one of the three 2-year, randomized, controlled trials of monthly intravitreal ranibizumab treatment (MARINA, ANCHOR or FOCUS trial). Of the 853 patients, two-year VA data were available for 384 [37]. These patients could receive 0.5 mg ranibizumab at 30-day or longer intervals as needed. Of the patients who received initial treatment with ranibizumab during the ANCHOR, MARINA, and FOCUS trials, there was a mean 10.2-letter increase in VA during the first 2 years of the studies Patients that did not receive anti-VEGF therapy in those trials had worse outcomes. During the first year of the HORIZON study and the third year of the original trials, there was a 5.1-letter loss The initial VA gain decreased by a mean of 8 letters with less frequent dosing in years 3 and 4. During the as needed dosing phase, the mean number of injections in the group initially treated with ranibizumab was 3.6. compared to 4.2 injections for patients that were treated with sham in the original trials.

The results of the HORIZON trial demonstrate that a delay in the initiation of treatment is associated with poorer visual outcomes and continued but less frequent dosing in years 3 and 4 was associated as well with visual decline [37].

PRN regimen of ranibizumab guided by monthly BCVA and other ophthalmic examinations, as detailed before, appears effective in sustaining the BCVA gained with 12 monthly injections with a significant lower number of injections during the extension phase [38].

Each one of these studies evaluated PRN regimens and had its own retreatment criteria, most of them retreated patients with a 100 μm increase in CRT from the thinnest measurement, and/or a Decreased VA >5 letters compared with VA score from the previous scheduled study visit, but each study had its particular criteria, and follow up regimen. All those studies mentioned previously have used the Time Domain OCT which is less accurate than the Spectral Domain OCT (SD-OCT) – therefore re-treatment criteria usually used the 100 microns increase in thickness. Nowadays by using the SD OCT, residual or recurrent fluid which is less than 100 microns in height can be detected, so patients are re-treated earlier – which may account for a better visual outcome using the PRN regimen. Strengths of PRONTO and SUSTAIN include monthly follow-up, but the PRONTO trialconsists of only a small cohort of patients. The SAILOR trial is the largest, but mandated only quarterly follow up visits. Overall, these studies support frequent follow up and individualized retreatment to achieve the best visual acuity gains with the as-needed treatment regimen as an alternative to the traditional monthly treatments used in the ANCHOR and MARINA trials. Furthermore, the CATT study (detailed later) showed that ranibizumab given as needed with monthly evaluation had effects on vision that were equivalent to those of ranibizumab administered monthly.

4.2. Ranibizumab: Treat-and-extend regimen

Treat-and-extend dosing regimen was first described by Freund et al. for the treatment of retinal angiomatous proliferation with an anti-VEGF agent. It involved increasing intervals between intravitreal injections up to 10 weeks as long as no fluid is present on OCT. If fluid is present, the interval between treatments is shortened[39].The treat-and-extend regimen is quite variable in terms of treatment criteria, which can include vision loss and/or macular hemorrhage [39], and the time between treatment, which can extend up to 12 weeks [40, 41]. Unfortunately, there are no large, randomized, prospective trials that investigated the efficacy of this regimen compared to the PRN protocol.

Oubraham et al. compared two ranibizumab retreatment strategies; as-needed (PRN) and treat-and-extend, in a retrospective review of 90 patients, 52 in the PRN group, and 38 in the treat-and-extend group. Their treatment regimen included 3 loading doses monthly for the first three months in both groups, and the decision to re-treat was based only on the existence of fluid on OCT They found that at one year, mean gain in VA was greater in the treat-and-extend group than in the PRN (+10.8 versus +2.3 letters, resp.). Eyes in the treat-and-extend group received significantly more injections (7.8 versus 5.2). Patients in the PRN group were followed every 4-5 weeks and the number of follow-up visits was similar in both groups (8.5 versus 8.8) [40].

Gupta et al. published a retrospective case series of 92 eyes treated with the treat-and-extend ranibizumab regimen. After 2 years, 32% had gained at least3 lines of vision and received 8.36 and 7.45 injections during the first and second years, respectively. In his study, this regimen was associated with fewer patient visits, injections, and direct annual medical costs compared with monthly injections [41].

4.3. Bevacizumab: As-needed regimen

The ABC trial is a prospective, double-masked, multicenter, randomized-controlled trial that included 131 patients randomized to 3 loading doses of bevacizumab at 6-week intervals followed by as-needed treatment at six week intervals or an alternate treatment atthe start of the trial (PDT, pegaptanib, or sham). Thirty-two percent of patients in the bevacizumab group gained at least15 letters with a mean VA increase of 7 letters vs a mean decrease of 9.4 letters in the alternate group. The median number of injections during the 12 months was 7 injections [42].

Other smaller, retrospective studies note a substantial improvement in VA using a protocol of three loading doses of bvacizumab followed by a PRN regimen, based mostly on OCT findings [43, 44].

Several retrospective studies demonstrated stabilization or improvement in VA following PRN treatment regimen with bevacizumab without a loading phase [45, 46]. One prospective, open-label, nonrandomized clinical study reported a mean VA gain of 8.6 letters in 51 eyes after their second year of PRN bevacizumab treatment with a mean of only 1.5injections given during year 2 [47].

4.4. Bevacizumab: Treat-and-extend regimen

Gupta et al. retrospectively reviewed 74 eyes of 73 patients with treatment-naive nvAMD. The patients were treated monthly with intravitreal bevacizumab until no intraretinal or subretinal fluid was observed on OCT. The treatment intervals then were lengthened sequentially by 2 weeks until signs of exudation recurred and then was reduced accordingly to maintain an exudation-free macula. Main outcomes measured included mean change from baseline visual acuity, proportion of eyes losing fewer than 3 and gaining 3 or more Snellen visual acuity lines at 1 year of follow-up, annual mean number of injections, OCT (Zeiss stratus) mean central retinal thickness change from baseline, mean maximum period of extension, adverse events, and mean direct annual medical cost. The mean follow-up period was 1.41 years. Mean Snellen VA improved from 20/230 at baseline to 20/109 at 12 months (P <.001) and 20/106 at 24 months (P <.001). The mean number of injections over the first year was 7.94. The mean OCT central retinal thickness decreased from 316 to 239 μm at 12 months (P <.001). The mean direct medical cost over the first year was $3493.85.

The treat and-extend regimen in their study, was associated with significant visual improvements with fewer patient visits and injections along with lower costs when compared to the MARINA, ANCHOR, and PrONTO protocols [48].

5. Comparison of AMD treatment trials (CATT and IVAN trials)

Several retrospective studies have tried to evaluate the efficacy of ranibizumab as compared to bevacizumab, however they were not powered enough to show the differences in efficacy or safety between the 2 drugs. The CATT and the IVAN trials are two prospective large scale randomized controlled trials that compared the two drugs in different regimens of treatment. The CATT trial is a multicenter, single-blind, non-inferiority trial that collectively enrolled 1208 patients with nvAMD [49]. Patients were randomized to 4 treatment groups: monthly bevacizumab, monthly ranibizumab, as-needed bevacizumab and as needed ranibizumab. In the as needed groups, retreatment was performed if at least one of the following criteria was met: fluid present on Time Domain OCT, decreased VA as compared to previous exam, new or persistent hemorrhage detected on clinical exam, or dye leakage or increased lesion size visible on fluorescein angiography. The primary outcome measure was mean change in VA at one year. The results at 12 months showed that Bevacizumab administered monthly was equivalent to ranibizumab administered monthly, with 8.0 and 8.5 letters gained, respectively. Bevacizumab administered as needed was equivalent to ranibizumab as needed, with 5.9 and 6.8 letters gained, respectively. Ranibizumab as needed was equivalent to monthly ranibizumab, although the comparison between bevacizumab as needed and monthly bevacizumab was inconclusive. Ranibizumab as-needed was found to be equivalent to monthly ranibizumab, but the comparison between bevacizumab as-needed and monthly ranibizumab was inconclusive [49]. This could be due to the less durable treatment effect of bevacizumab in a subgroup of patients [50]. Ranibizumab given as needed was equivalent to bevacizumab given monthly. The comparison between bevacizumab given as needed and ranibizumab given monthly was also inconclusive.

The mean decrease in central retinal thickness was greater in the ranibizumab-monthly group (196 μm) than in the other groups (152 to 168 μm, P=0.03 by analysis of variance) Although not powered sufficiently to compare adverse event rates associated with the two drugs, the rates of death, arteriothrombotic events, and venous thrombotic events were similar for patients receiving bevacizumab or ranibizumab. The rate of serious systemic adverse events, primarily hospitalizations, was higher among the patients who had received bevacizumab, but rates of adverse events did not increase with increased exposure to the drug [49].

At 1 year, patients initially assigned to monthly treatment were reassigned randomly to monthly or as-needed treatment, without changing the drug assignment[51] The 2 year results demonstrate that among patients receiving monthly injections for 2 years, mean gain in visual acuity was similar for both drugs (bevacizumab-ranibizumab difference, -1.4 letters; 95% confidence interval [CI], -3.7 to 0.8; P = 0.21). However mean gain was greater for monthly than for as-needed treatment (difference, -2.4 letters; 95% CI, -4.8 to -0.1; P = 0.046). The proportion of patients without fluid on OCT ranged from 13.9% in the bevacizumab-as-needed group to 45.5% in the ranibizumab monthly group (drug, P = 0.0003; regimen, P < 0.0001). Switching from monthly to as-needed treatment in the second year resulted in greater mean decrease in vision during year 2 (-2.2 letters; P = 0.03) and a lower proportion without fluid (-19%; P < 0.0001). Rates of death and arteriothrombotic events were similar for both drugs (P > 0.60). The proportion of patients with 1 or more systemic serious adverse events was higher with bevacizumab than ranibizumab (39.9% vs. 31.7%; adjusted risk ratio, 1.30; 95% CI, 1.07-1.57; P = 0.009), even thoughmost of the excess events have not been associated previously with systemic therapy targeting vascular endothelial growth factor (VEGF) [51].

The first year results from an NIHR Health Technology Assessment (HTA) programmed funded trial, IVAN (Inhibit VEGF in Age related choroidal Neovascularization) were recently published [52]. The trial compared the efficacy of ranibizumab vs bevacizumab in 610 subjects with nvAMD from 23 hospitals and academic institutions in the UK. In addition blood samples were repeatedly evaluated for the VEGF concentration in the plasma. Patients received injections of the drug into the affected eye every month for the first three months. Groups were then subdivided to receive either injections at every visit thereafter namely the continuous group or only if the specialist decided there was persistent disease – namely the discontinuous group. Whenever re-treatment was performed the patient received a series of 3 monthly consecutive injections as opposed to 1 injection given in the CATT. After 12 months the comparison between the two drugs was inconclusive (-1.99 letters in favor of the Ranibizumab, 95% confidence interval [CI], -4.04 to 0.06). Discontinuous treatment was equivalent to continuous treatment (-0.35 letters; 95% CI, -2.40 to 1.70). Mena foveal total thickness did not differ by drug, but was 9% less using the continuous treatment (geometric mean ratio [GMR], 0.91; 95% CI, 0.86 to 0.97; P = 0.005). Fewer participants receiving bevacizumab had an arteriothrombotic event or heart failure (odds ratio [OR], 0.23; 95% CI, 0.05 to 1.07; P = 0.03). There was no difference between drugs in the proportion of subjects experiencing a serious systemic adverse event (OR, 1.35; 95% CI, 0.80 to 2.27; P = 0.25). Serum VEGF levels were found to be significantly lower in subjects treated with bevacizuamb compared to ranibizumab (GMR, 0.47; 95% CI, 0.41 to 0.54; P<0.0001) and higher with discontinuous treatment compared to continuous treatment (GMR, 1.23; 95% CI, 1.07 to 1.42; P = 0.004). These results clearly indicate the higher systemic exposure to bevacizumab compared with ranibizumab. Researchers concluded that the comparison of VA at 1 year between bevacizumab and ranibizumab was inconclusive. Visual acuities with continuous and discontinuous treatment were equivalent. Other outcomes are consistent with the drugs and treatment regimens having similar efficacy and safety.

The results of the second year of the IVAN trial and others like the VIBERA (Germany), EQUAL (Netherlands) and MANTA (Austria) studies [53-55] are about to be published in the coming future.

6. Management of nonresponders

As many as 10% of patients demonstrate a significant loss of vision in spite of 2 years of monthly anti-VEGF therapy [9, 20]. Within this group of individuals exist those who progress to disciform scar, RPE tear, massive subretinal hemorrhage, geographic atrophy, and in addition eyes that demonstrate persistent macular fluid/blood and leakage on OCT and fluorescein angiography associated with vision loss. This subgroup of patients is referred to as anti-VEGF non-responders. This variability in anti-VEGF treatment response can be attributed to more aggressive forms of nvAMD, including retinal angiomatous proliferation (RAP), tachyphylaxis to anti-VEGF drugs, mimics of wet AMD [56], and genetic differences among patients [57, 58].

The therapeutic approach in these patients include alternating bevacizumab and ranibizumab, switching to a newer anti VEGF drug- Eylea, combination therapy which is further discussed in the next section, or other treatment options such as brachytherapy and transpupillary thermotherapy.

6.1. Combination therapy

Since the development and progression of nvAMD involve pro-angiogenic factors, vascular permeability molecules, and inflammatory proteins, targeting only one component of this process may be insufficient and temporary, as shown by the data presented above. Anti VEGF agents are very effective in halting vascular leakage, but it has shown to be a temporizing treatment, and there is an increased need for a treatment with longer efficacy duration..The ideal combination therapy regimen would provide a longer-lasting treatment effect in addition to potentially being more or equally efficacious to monotherapy alone.

The main combination therapies are further discussed.

6.1.1. PDT+ anti VEGF

SUMMIT is a clinical trial program that includes three similarly designed, controlled studies to further examine the safety, efficacy, and treatment burden of combination therapy with PDT and ranibizumab compared with ranibizumab alone: DENALI in the USA, and Canada, examining verteporfin PDT in combination at both standard- and reduced-fluence light doses; MONT BLANC in Europe, examining verteporfin PDT in combination at standard-fluence light dose only, and an Asian study (EVEREST) which is designed to compare standard fluence PDT combined with ranibizumab and ranibizumab monotherapy in the treatment of polypoidal choroidal vasculopathy (PCV). Twelve-month results of the MONTBLANC study showed that combining standard-fluence PDT with ranibizumab 0.5mg results in VA improvement that is noninferior to a ranibizumab monotherapy regimen with three ranibizumab-loading doses followed by injections on a monthly PRN basis (non-inferiority margin of 7 letters There was no significant difference between the two treatment arms with regard to proportion of patients with a treatment-free interval of at least three months duration after month 2. Adverse event incidence was similar between treatment groups [59].As monotherapy is not inferior to the combination; they concluded that monotherapy should be the preferred treatment.

Twelve-month results of the DENALI study showed that combining PDT with ranibizumab in a regimen that consists three ranibizumab loading doses followed by additional injections on a monthly PRN basis and PRN PDT every 3 months can improve VA at month 12 in patients with sub foveal CNV secondary to nvAMD [60]. However the combination treatment was found inferior to the monotherapy with ranibizumab alone. At month 12, patients in the standard fluence combination group and the reduced fluence combination group gained on average 5.3 and 4.4 letters from baseline, compared to a more significant gain of 8.1 letters in the ranibizumab monthly monotherapy group. DENALI did not demonstrate non-inferior visual acuity gain for PDT combination therapy compared with ranibizumab monthly monotherapy, meaning the monotherapy with monthly ranibizumab was found superior to the combination therapy.

Six months results of the EVEREST trial were recently published [61]. At Month 6, verteporfin PDT combined with ranibizumab or verteporfin PDT alone was superior to ranibizumab monotherapy in achieving complete polyp regression (77.8% and 71.4% vs. 28.6%; $P < 0.01$); mean change ± standard deviation in best-corrected visual acuity (letters) was the highest in the combination group although not statistically better than the ranibizumab monotherapy. There was a mean improvement of 10.9 ± 10.9 letters in the verteporfin PDT + ranibizumab, 7.5 ± 10.6 letters in the verteporfin PDT alone, and 9.2 ± 12.4 letters in the ranibizumab monotherapy. There were no new safety findings with either drug used alone or in combination. Based on the results of the EVERST we can conclude that combination therapy of reduced fluence PDT with ranibizumab should be applied in cases of PCV, because this combined treatment yields the best VA results and highest rate of anatomic closure of the polyps.

6.1.2. Triple therapy

Augustin et al. described a combination therapy involving standard fluence PDT with reduced light duration (70 seconds instead of 83 seconds),with total light dose of 42J/ cm2. Sixteen hours after PDT administration patients were taken to the operating room, and underwent limited vitrectomy followed by intravitreal dexamethasone (800 mcg) and intravitreal bevacizumab (1.5 mg) injections [62]. Most patients treated with this triple therapy hadlong-lasting improvement in VA with only one treatment at final follow-up (The mean follow-up period was 40 weeks (range, 22-60 weeks). Less than one-fourth of the patients treated with this regimen required additional treatment either with repeat triple therapy or anti-VEGF alone during the follow-up period [62].

Bakri et al. retrospectively reviewed the treatment benefit in patients receiving a same-day combination of reduced fluence PDT, intravitreal dexamethasone (200mcg), and intravitreal bevacizumab (1.25 mg). Patients were either treatment naïve or previously treated. At final follow-up, patients treated with this regimen showed stable VA and decreased macular thickness [63].

An average of less than one additional treatment with either repeat triple therapy or anti-VEGF was required in the treatment of naive group while almost four additional treatments were required in previously treated patients [63]. No steroid-related complications were noted in either study [62, 63]. A prospective interventional case series of 17 patients treated with a same-day regimen of standard fluence PDT, intravitreal bevacizumab(1.25 mg), and intravitreal triamcinolone (IVTA) (2 mg), was recently published. Patients treated with this regimen also showed an improvement in VA and reduced central macular thickness [64].

The Reduced Fluence Visudyne Anti-VEGF Dexamethasone in Combination for AMD Lesions (RADICAL) trial is a prospective, multicenter, randomized trial of combination therapy for the treatment of wet AMD that began in 2008. Patients are randomized into four treatment arms including anti-VEGF monotherapy with ranibizumab, half-fluence PDT with ranibizumab, half-fluence PDT with ranibizumab and dexamethasone, or quarter-fluence PDT with ranibizumab and dexamethasone. The dose of ranibizumab used was 0.5 mg and dexamethasone 500 mcg. Patients enrolled in the trial were followed for a total of 24 months. For the first 12 months, patients were followed monthly with decision for retreatment made at each visit. After 12 months, patients were reassessed every 3 months or sooner at physician's discretion. Patients in the anti-VEGF monotherapy arm received mandatory first 3 monthly consecutive injections followed by retreatment as needed thereafter. Retreatment with combination therapy was not administered prior to 8 weeks interval. Twelve-month data released by the sponsor [65], QLT incorporated, showed significantly fewer re-treatments in all combination therapy arms compared with the groups of patients treated with anti-VEGF monotherapy [65].

VA appears to equally improve among all groups, but confidence intervals varied. Of the three combination therapy arms, the triple therapy half-fluence PDT group shared similar mean visual improvement compared with monotherapy and had the fewest re-treatments. After 12 months, three retreatments of triple therapy with half-fluence PDT were required compared to 5.1 re-treatments of monotherapy ($p<0.001$). Adverse event incidence was similar amongst all treatment groups. The final results of the 24-months trial were not published yet.

7. Potential complications of anti VEGF agents

Safety issues with anti VEGF intravitreal injections include local ocular adverse events (AEs) from the drug or the injection, as well as potential systemic AEs of the drug.

Ocular AEs may be categorized as common but not serious and rare but potentially serious. The AEs that are considered common but not serious include subconjunctival hemorrhage, vitreous floaters from medication or vitreous hemorrhage, and discomfort from antiseptic used to prepare the conjunctiva before the injection(9, 20, 21).

Repeated intravitreal injection of ranibizumab or bevacizumab, over extended time periods, has been demonstrated to result in a low incidence of serious ocular adverse events. In the CATT study, endophthalmitis developed after only two of 5449 injections (0.04%) in 599 patients treated with ranibizumab, and after only four of 5508 injections (0.07%) in 586 patients treated with bevacizumab. Uveitis, retinal detachment, retinal vascular occlusion or embolism, retinal tear, and vitreous hemorrhage each also occurred in less than 1% of patients [49, 50]. Efforts are underway in order to further reduce the incidence of these events, with studies evaluating the effect of needle type and injection technique on patient pain levels, vitreal reflux, and ocular complications [66].

It is unknown if pretreatment antibiotics for several days prior to injection, or only on the procedure's day is necessary in order to reduce the risk of endophthalmitis. Furthermore, it is unknown if post treatment antibiotics are necessary on the day of the procedure or thereafter to reduce this risk furthermore. Although the product insert for ranibizumab indicates that the administration of the intravitreal injection should include the use of sterile gloves and a sterile drape, not all physicians agree that these items are necessary to maintain sterile conditions for the injection. However, all agree that the use of a lid speculum and administration of povidone-iodine to the lids, lashes, and conjunctiva are recommended [67].

Another concern is an allergic reaction to the drug. Since ranibizumab is a recombinant monoclonal antibody that contains both mouse and human derived segments, some patients treated with the drug may develop systemic antibodies [8, 20].

In the ANCHOR trial 3.9% of ranibizumab 0.5-mg subjects had developed antibodies to ranibizumab compared with 0% in the PDT group [20].

In the MARINA trial, after 24 months, 6.3% of subjects treated with ranibizumab 0.5 mg and 1.1% of those in the sham injection group developed antibodies to ranibizumab [8].

Systemic AEs are a concern, since inhibitors of VEGF injected intravitreally, can penetrate the general circulation and compromise functions that rely on VEGF outside of the eye, such as wound healing and the formation of new blood vessels around the heart or brain in cases of ischemia [68, 69]. Patients with AMD already are at higher risk of cardiovascular disease than the general population because of their age and the association of AMDwith systemic hypertension [70], consequently, participants in clinical trialsof VEGF inhibitors were carefully monitored for possible increases in blood pressure, occurrence of myocardial infarction/stroke, and nonocular hemorrhages [8, 20].

Among participants in the MARINA trial, approximately16% in both the ranibizumab 0.5 mg and sham injectiongroups developed hypertension [8] and in the ANCHOR treatment related hypertension was higher in the PDT group (8.4%) than in the ranibizumab group (6.4%) [20].

In the CATT trial there was no evidence that ranibizumab0.5 mg was associated with increases in either diastolic or systolic blood pressure [49, 50].

Nonocular hemorrhages include events such as cerebral or gastrointestinal bleeding. In the ANCHOR trial, non ocular hemorrhage was more frequent in the 0.5-mg ranibizumab group (6.4%) than in the PDT group (2.1%) [20]. In the MARINA trial, the cumulative frequency of nonocular hemorrhage by month 24 was 5.5% in the sham injection group compared with 8.8% in the 0.5-mgranibizumab group [8].

Among participants in the MARINA trial, approximately 16% in both the ranibizumab 0.5 mg and sham injection groups developed hypertension [3].

In the CATT trial Gastrointestinal disorders (e.g., hemorrhage, hernia, nausea, and vomiting), occurred in 11 (1.8%) ranibizumab-treated and in 28 (4.8%) bevacizumab-treated patients ($P = 0.005$) [51].

With respect to cardiovascular or cerebrovascular events, during the ANCHOR trial, 1 subject in the PDT group (0.7%) and 3 subjects in the ranibizumab 0.5-mg group (2.1%) developed nonfatal myocardial infarctions, although the events did not occurshortly after treatment. [20]. The frequency of stroke (1 in each group) and cerebral infarction (0 in each group) in the ANCHOR trial were too low to draw meaningful conclusion [20].

At 24 months, the overall frequency of cardiovascular systemic events in the MARINA trial was similar in the0.5-mg ranibizumab and sham injection groups [8]. Therewere only small differences in the frequency of thromboembolic events between the sham injection group (3.8%) and the ranibizumab 0.5-mg group (4.6%) [8]. The frequency of death (2.5%) was the same in the ranibizumab 0.5-mgand sham injection groups [8]. Two individuals in each group died of stroke.

There was no significant difference in the frequency of myocardial infarction between the 2 treatment groups in the SAILOR trial [36].

In the CATT trial at 2 years, 5.3% assigned to ranibizumab and 6.1% assigned to Bevacizumab had died ($P = 0.62$). The proportion of patients with arteriothrombotic events was similar in the ranibizumab-treated patients (4.7%) and in the bevacizumab-treated patients 5.0%; (P = 0.89). Venous thrombotic events occurred in 3 (0.5%) ranibizumab-treated patients and in 10 (1.7%) bevacizumab-treated patients (P = 0.054) [51].

One or more serious systemic adverse events occurred in 255 patients (21.5%), with 53 (17.6%) in the ranibizumab-monthly group, 64 (22.4%) in the bevacizumab-monthly group, 61 (20.5%) in the ranibizumab-as-needed group, and 77 (25.7%) in the bevacizumab-as-needed group (P = 0.11 by the chi-square test). Hospitalizations accounted for 298 of the 370 individual serious systemic adverse events (80.5%). When dosing-regimen groups were combined, the proportions of patients with serious systemic adverse events were 24.1% for bevacizumab and 19.0% for ranibizumab (P = 0.04). After adjustment for demographic features and coexisting illnesses at baseline, the risk ratio for bevacizumab, as compared with ranibizumab, was 1.29 (95% confidence interval, 1.01 to 1.66; P = 0.04). Patients treated as needed had higher rates than patients treated monthly (risk ratio, 1.20; 95% CI, 0.98–1.47; P =0.08). After excluding all events previously associated with systemic treatment with anti–vascular endothelial growth factor drugs, 170 (28.4%) of ranibizumab-treated patients and 202 (34.5%) of bevacizumab-treated patients had experienced events (P = 0.02) [51].

Although event rates for these cerebrovascular or cardiovascular events seem to be low with ranibizumab, ophthalmologists should ensure that patients understand the theoretic potential for these risks. Additional studies over time may help to refine understanding of the magnitude, if any, of this risk.

In the recently published IVAN trial at 12 months, 6 participants (1.9%) in the ranibizumab group and 5 (1.7%) in the bevacizumab group (P = 0.81) had died; 5 (1.6%) had received continuous and 6 (2.0%) discontinuous treatment (P = 0.74) [52]. Fewer participants treated with bevacizumab compared with ranibizumab had an arteriothrombotic event or heart failure (0.7% vs. 2.9%; odds ratio, 0.23; 95% CI, 0.05to 1.07; P = 0.03), but no difference between treatment regimens was found (P = 0.34). One or more serious systemic adverse events occurred in 30 (9.6%) in the ranibizumab group and 37 (12.5%) in the bevacizumab group (P = 0.25). Similarly, 30 (9.7%) in the continuous and 7 (12.3%) in the discontinuous group had ≥1 serious systemic adverse events (P = 0.32). More than 10 participant-specific events occurred in 3 MedDRA categories: cardiac disorders, surgical or medical procedure, and any other class (available at http://aaojournal.org). Comparisons by drug and regimen for cardiac disorders and surgical or medical procedure showed no differences (P≥0.46). One case of severe uveitis developed after 1 injection; there was 1 reported traumatic cataract and 3 retinal pigment epithelial tears. Five "other" ocular events were each reported once.

7.1. Safety of Bevacizumab

Data on the safety of intravitreal bevacizumab are more limited than data on Ranibizumab safety, due to the lack of large multicenter trials performed with Bevacizumab. The results of the CATT and IVAN trials were previously presented.

8. New anti VEGF agents under investigation

8.1. RNA Interference (SIRNA)

SIRNA stands for short interfering RNA. SIRNAs are 21 to 25 nucleotide-long double-stranded RNA molecules capable of destroying a corresponding target messenger RNA with high selectivity and efficacy [71]. This leads to post transcriptional gene silencing (PTGS).

SIRNAs work intracellularly, where they are incorporated into a protein complex called RNA-induced silencing complex (RISC) [71]. The RISC has RNA helicase activity, which unwinds the two strands of RNA. The strand of the siRNA that becomes associated to the RISC leads the complex to selectively cleave and degrade messenger RNA molecules containing a complementary sequence. The siRNA is engineered to match the protein encoding nucleotide sequence of the target messenger RNA. Since the translation of messenger RNA into proteins is an amplification step, destroying it is a very potent method of inhibiting protein function.

SIRNA-027 (SIRNA Therapeutics, Inc.) is a short interfering RNA that targets the VEGF receptor 1 (VEGFR-1).Animal experiments have shown that both intravitreous and periocular injections of siRNA directed against VEGFR1 lead to a substantial reduction of VEGFR1 messenger RNA levels [71-72].

The siRNA suppressed the development of CNV at rupture sites in Bruch's membrane and decreased retinal neovascularizationin mice with oxygen-induced ischemic retinopathy [72-73].

Acuity Pharmaceuticals has also produced a siRNA called Cand5 or Bevasiranib that targets the messenger RNA of the VEGF protein itself. Animal models have shown prevention of CNV development after laser-induced injury [72].

Bevasiranib sodium was developed for intravitreal administration. Following intravitreal injection, bevasiranib is well distributed within the eye and localizes to the retina [72, 73].

Preliminary results of Phases I and II clinical trials of bevasiranib have shown promising results for the treatment of nvAMD and diabetic macular edema. There are various studies of different phases underway (the COBALT studies although recruitment was stopped). A phase III study evaluating the combination of bevasiranib and ranibizumab in nvAMD (the CARBON study) is currently underway.

The purpose of this study is to compare intravitreal bevasiranib sodium as maintenance therapy for AMD following initiation with three monthly doses of ranibizumab. Preliminary clinical results indicate that the effects of bevasiranib do not appear until six weeks after the initiation of treatment, which suggests that combination therapy with anti VEGF drug might be justified. The late effect of bevasiranib might be linked to its mechanism of action, since bevasiranib inhibits the synthesis of new VEGF, and does not eliminate existing VEGF, a direct anti-VEGF agent may be required to neutralize VEGF already present in the eye before inhibition of new VEGF synthesis. Preliminary results of the carbon and cobalt studies suggested that over 30% of patients on combination ranibizumab-bevasiranib achieve an improvement of at least three additional lines of VA than those on ranibizumab alone. The safety and efficacy of this combination awaits the full results of the ongoing clinical trials.

However, the lack of available data from randomized placebo-controlled or comparative studies makes it difficult to evaluate the role of bevasiranib in nvAMD therapy. It is clear from experimental and preclinical studies that anti-VEGF siRNA is capable of down regulating VEGF production, a key goal of anti-VEGF therapy [72].

In summary, bevasiranib exploits an interesting technology [72, 73] and may be a useful addition to the currently available drugs used to treat wet AMD.

8.2. Tyrosine kinase inhibitors

VEGF A signals through two VEGF receptors [7, 10]. VEGF R consist of protein-tyrosine kinases (VEGFR-1, VEGFR-2, and VEGFR-3) and two non-protein kinase coreceptors (neuropilin-1 and neuropilin-2) [10]. New drugs targeting these tyrosine kinases are being investigated.

Vatalanib (PTK787; Novartis)- Vatalanib [74] is a potent tyrosine kinase inhibitor with good oral bioavailability and activity against the VEGFR family, PDGFRβ and c-Kit receptor kinases. Preclinical studies [74] suggest that vatalanib induces dose-dependent inhibition of VEGF-induced angiogenesis. A phase I/II trial, ADVANCE [75], to evaluate the safety and efficacy of oral vatalanib combined with PDT with verteporfin in 50 patients has been completed, but the data have not yet been published in a peer-reviewed journal.

Pazopanib (GW786034; GlaxoSmithKline)- Pazopanib [76] is a second-generation tyrosine kinase inhibitor against all VEGFR, PDGFRα, PDGFRβ, and c-kit. A phase I clinical trial using pazopanib as eye drops in 38 healthy volunteers has successfully demonstrated its safety and tolerability. Subsequently, a phase II trial [77] to evaluate its pharmacodynamics, pharmacokinetics and safety has been completed, but the data have not yet been published in a peer-reviewed journal.

8.3. Anti-VEGFR vaccine therapy

This is an immunologic approach to combat CNV. A recent report demonstrated CD8+ cytotoxic T lymphocyte (CTL)-mediated regression of physiologic and pathologic retinal neovascularization [78], thus a possible immunologic therapy for CNV was suggested. It was approved by an animal model [79] which showed that CNV can regress by inducing cellular immunity specific for VEGFR-2.

More recently, a phase I study [80] of anti-VEGFR vaccine therapy has been recruiting participants. The patients will be vaccinated once a week for 12 weeks. On each vaccination day, VEGFR-1 peptide (1 mg) and VEGFR-2 peptide (1 mg) mixed with Montanide ISA 51 will be administered by subcutaneous injection. The study will evaluate the safety and tolerability as well as the immunological and clinical response of the vaccine therapy to treatment of nvAMD.

http://dx.doi.org/10.5772/54198

8.4. Anti inflammatory mediators

As mentioned before, both angiogenic and inflammatory processes are involved in nvAMD, new therapeutics targeting the inflammatory process, besides steroids are being investigated

POT-4 (Potentia Pharmaceuticals)- POT-4 [81] is a peptide capable of binding to human complement factor C3 (C3). As C3 is a central component of all known complement activation pathways, its inhibition effectively shuts down all downstream complement activation that could otherwise lead to local inflammation, tissue damage and up-regulation of angiogenic factors such as VEGF.

A phase I single escalating dose study [82] has just released its first results, which indicate that POT-4 IVT is safe, and the data accumulated so far support the continued investigation of POT-4 for the treatment of both dry and wet AMD with a larger randomized phase II trial to further define its efficacy profile.

ARC1905 (Ophthotech Corp.) -ARC1905 [81] is an anti-C5 aptamer, which prevents the formation of key terminal fragments (C5a and C5b-9) by inhibiting human complement factor C5 (C5). C5a fragment is an important inflammatory activator inducing vascular permeability, recruitment and activation of phagocytes. C5b-9 is involved in the formation of membrane attack complex (C5b-9), which initiates cell lysis [81]. Thus by inhibiting these C5-mediated inflammatory, ARC1905 might be beneficial in wet AMD.

A phase I study [83] to evaluate the safety, tolerability, and pharmacokinetic profile of multiple doses of ARC1905 IVT in combination with multiple doses of Lucentis has been completed, but the data have not yet been published in a peer-reviewed journal.

OT-551 (Othera)-OT-551 [84], an Othera Pharmaceuticals' Othera (OT)-551 antioxidant eye drop has the potential for chronic treatment of the dry form of age-related macular degeneration.

A phase I trial [84] demonstrated that when the compound is added to Lucentis or Avastin treatment, there is a synergistic effect in patients with wet AMD. A pilot study [85] of participants with bilateral geographic atrophy is designed to characterize the effect of 0.45% concentration of OT-551 eye drops on the progression of geographic atrophy area over a two-year period.

8.5. AdPEDF - Fovista (GenVec)

Pigment epithelium-derived factor (PEDF) is one of the most potent antiangiogenic proteins found in humans, which were shown to inhibit VEGF-induced proliferation, migration of microvascular endothelial cells, reduce VEGF-induced hypermeability and cause vessel regression in established neovascularization [86]. AdPEDF uses a DNA carrier, to deliver the PEDF gene, resulting in the local production of AdPEDF in the treated eye.

A phase I escalating-dose clinical trial [87] in patients with nvAMD was completed. Three to six months after a single injection, it suggested that 50–94% of patients had a stabilization or improvement in lesion size from baseline, suggesting that antiangiogenesis may last for several months after a single IVT. there were no dose-limiting toxicities or drug-related severe adverse events reported. Further studies investigating the efficacy of AdPEDF in patients with wet AMD are under way.

Trial	No. of patients	Injection protocol	Drug, dosage, control	Results
VISION	1186	IVT every 6 weeks	Pegaptanib; 0.3/1.0/3.0 mg-Sham	31%–37% stable vision, 4%–6%gained "/>3 lines (12 months)
MARINA	716	IVT monthly	Ranibizumab; 0.3/0.5 mg-sham	95% stable vision, 26%–34% gained"/>3 lines (12 months)
ANCHOR	423	IVT monthly	Ranibizumab; 0.3/0.5 mg-Sham + PDT every 3 months if needed	96%Stable vision,35%–40% gained"/>3lines (12 months)
FOCUS	162	IVT monthly+PDT	Ranibizumab; 0.5 mg-PDT every 3 months	90% stable vision
HORIZON	853	IVT monthly	Ranibizumab; 0.5 mg	Mean loss of vision 2–5 letters, 3% gained "/>3 lines, 7%–14% lost "/>3 lines (12 months)
PIER	183	IVT monthly x 3, re-treatment every 3 months	Ranibizumab; 0.3/0.5 mg-sham	83%–90% stable vision, 12%–13% gained "/ >3lines (12 months)
PRONTO	37	IVT monthly x 3, re-treatment as needed (9.9 injections over 24 months)	Ranibizumab; 0.5 mg	43% gained "/>3 lines (24 months)
SUSTAIN	513	IVT monthly x 3, re treatment as needed (5.3 injections for "naïve" patients over 12 months)	Ranibizumab; 0.3/0.5 mg	Mean BCVA increased steadily from baseline to month 3 to reach +5.8 letters, decreased slightly from month 3 to 6, and remained stable from month 6 to 12, reaching +3.6 at month 12
CLEAR-IT	51	IVT single	Aflibercept; 0.05/0.15/0.5/1.0/2.0/4 .0 mg	95% stable vision, 50% of 2.0/4.0 mg group gained "/>3 lines (3 months)
VIEW1 VIEW2	1217 1240	VTE 0.5 mg monthly (0.5q4wk), VTE 2 mg monthly (2q4wk),VTE 2 mg every two months (2q8wk), or ranibizumab 0.5mg monthly (Rq4wk)	Aflibercept (VTE);0.5/2.0 mg-Ranibizumab;0.5 mg	All VTE groups were noninferior to ranibizumab.

Table 1. Summary of main clinical trials on anti VEGF treatment for AMD

http://dx.doi.org/10.5772/54198

9. Conclusion

Over the past decade, the treatment of nvAMD improved dramatically with the discovery of anti-VEGF agents that have enabled patients not only to stabilize the vision but to improve and regain vision in this potentially blinding disease.

With the goal of maximizing VA and minimizing the frequency of intravitreal injections and associated risks of treatment, evidence-based management of wet AMD has evolved into individualized anti-VEGF therapy with frequent follow up and retreatment. As a safer and more cost-effective alternative to the traditional monthly treatments used in the ANCHOR and MARINA trials, two individualized anti-VEGF treatment regimens have been described, but neither has been proven superior to date: as-needed (or "PRN") therapy and the treat-and-extend strategy. Despite a paucity of evidence comparing the as-needed versus the treat-and extend treatment regimens, a possibility exists that the treat and extend regimen will prove to be the most efficacious, cost-saving, and preferred protocol. The current evidence based treatment strategy for the management of wet AMD supports the use of either bevacizumab or ranibizumab either monthly or with a more individualized treatmentstrategy with close followup. As second generation anti-VEGF agents become available and the stress on our healthcaresystems intensifies, increasingly efficacious and costconscioustreatment strategies will be essential.

Author details

Shani Golan[1,2], Michaella Goldstein[1,2] and Anat Loewenstein[1,2]

1 Department of Ophthalmology Tel Aviv Medical Center, Israel

2 Sackler Faculty of Medicine, Tel Aviv University, Tel- Aviv, Israel

References

[1] Alm A. Ocular circulation. In: Hart WM, editor. Adler's Physiology of the Eye. St Louis, USA: Mosby Year Book; 1992. p. 198 – 227.

[2] Folkman J, Ingber D. Inhibition of angiogenesis. Semin Cancer Biol. 1992;3:89 – 96.

[3] J. Z. Nowak, "Age-related macular degeneration (AMD): pathogenesis and therapy," Pharmacological Reports, vol. 58, no. 3, pp. 353–363, 2006.

[4] Smith W, Assink J, Klein R, Mitchell P, Klaver CCW,Klein BEK, et al. Risk factors for age-related macular degeneration: Pooled fi ndings from three continents. Ophthalmology. 2001;108:697 – 704.

[5] Kinnunen K, Ylä-Herttuala S. Vascular endothelial growth factors in retinal and choroidal neovascular disease. Ann Med. 2012 Feb;44(1):1-17

[6] Shima DT, Nishijima K, Jo N, Adamis AP. VEGF-mediated neuroprotectionin ischemic retinal.Invest Ophthalmol Vis Sci. 2004;45:3270

[7] Terman BI, Dougher-Vermazen M, Carrion ME et al. Identification of the KDR tyrosine kinase as a receptor for vascular endothelial growth factor. Biochem Biophys Res Commun. 1992;187:1579-86.

[8] Ciulla TA, Rosenfeld PJ. Antivascular endothelial growth factor therapy for neovascular age-related macular degeneration. Curr Opin Ophthalmol. 2009 May;20(3): 158-65.

[9] Rosenfeld PJ, Brown DM, Heier JS, Boyer DS, Kaiser PK,hung CY, et al. Ranibizumab for neovascular age-relatedacular degeneration. N Engl J Med. 2006;355:1419 – 31.

[10] H. Yonekura, S. Sakurai, X. Liu et al., "Placenta growth factor and vascular endothelial growth factor B and C expression in microvascular endothelial cells and pericytes. Implication in autocrine and paracrine regulation of angiogenesis," Journal of Biological Chemistry, vol. 274, no. 49, pp. 35172–35178, 1999.

[11] H. Takahashi and M. Shibuya, "The vascular endothelial growth factor (VEGF)/ VEGF receptor system and its role under physiological and pathological conditions," Clinical Science, vol. 109, no. 3, pp. 227–241, 2005.

[12] X. Yi, N. Ogata, M. Komada et al., "Vascular endothelial growth factor expression in choroidal neovascularization in rats," Graefe's Archive for Clinical and Experimental Ophthalmology, vol. 235, no. 5, pp. 313–319, 1997.

[13] B. A. Keyt, L. T. Berleau, H. V. Nguyen et al., "The carboxylterminal domain (111–165) of vascular endothelial growth factor is critical for its mitogenic potency," Journal of Biological Chemistry, vol. 271, no. 13, pp. 7788–7795, 1996.

[14] S. Ishida, T. Usui, K. Yamashiro et al., "VEGF164-mediated inflammation is required for pathological, but not physiological, ischemia-induced retinal neovascularization," Journal of Experimental Medicine, vol. 198, no. 3, pp. 483–489, 2003.

[15] A. Kvanta, P. V. Algvere, L. Berglin, and S. Seregard, "Subfoveal fibrovascular membranes in age-related macular degeneration express vascular endothelial growth factor," Investigative Ophthalmology and Visual Science, vol. 37, no. 9, pp. 1929–1934, 1996.

[16] D 'A mico DJ. Pegaptanib sodium for neovascular age related macular degeneration: two-year safety results of the two prospective, multicenter, controlled clinical trials. Ophthalmology. 2006;113:992 – 1001.

[17] Gragoudas ES, Adamis AP, Cunningham ET Jr, Feinsod M, Guyer DR; VEGF Inhibition Study in Ocular Neovascularization Clinical Trial Group. Pegaptanib for neovascular age-related macular degeneration. N Engl J Med. 2004 Dec 30;351(27):2805-16.

[18] VEGF Inhibition Study in Ocular Neovascularization (V.I.S.I.O.N.) Clinical Trial Group, Chakravarthy U, Adamis AP, Cunningham ET Jr, Goldbaum M, Guyer DR, Katz B, Patel M. Year 2 efficacy results of 2 randomized controlled clinical trials of pegaptanib for neovascular age-related macular degeneration. Ophthalmology. 2006 Sep;113(9):1508.e1-25.

[19] N. Feucht, H. Matthias, C. P. Lohmann, and M. Maier "Pegaptanib sodium treatment in neovascular age-related macular degeneration: clinical experience in Germany," Clinical Ophthalmology, vol. 2, pp. 253–259, 2008.

[20] Brown DM, Michels M, Kaiser PK, Heier JS, Sy JP, Ianchulev T; ANCHOR Study Group. Ranibizumab versus verteporfin photodynamic therapy for neovascular age-related macular degeneration: Two-year results of the ANCHOR study.Ophthalmology. 2009 Jan;116(1):57-65.e5.

[21] Regillo CD, Brown DM, Abraham P et al. Randomized, double-masked, sham controlledtrial of ranibizumab for neovascular age-relatedmacular degeneration: PIER study year 1. Am J Ophthalmol.2008;145:239 – 48.

[22] U. Schmidt-Erfurth, B. Eldem, R. Guymer et al., "Efficacy and safety of monthly versus quarterly ranibizumab treatment inneovascular age-related macular degeneration. The EXCITE study," Ophthalmology, vol. 118, pp. 831–839, 2010.

[23] Fung AE, Rosenfeld PJ, Reichel E. The international intravitreal bevacizumab safety survey: using the Internet to assess drug safety worldwide. Br J Ophthalmol 2007; 90:1344–1349.

[24] Schmidt-Erfurth UM, Pruente C. Management of neovascularage-related macular degeneration. Prog Retin Eye Res. 2007;26:437 – 51.

[25] Mordenti J, Cuthbertson RA, Ferrara N et al . Comparisons of the intraocular tissue distribution, pharmacokinetics and safety of 1251-labeled full-length and Fab antibodies in rhesus monkeys following intravitreal administration. Toxicol Pathol 1999; 27:536-44.

[26] Shahar J, Avery RL, Heilweil G et al. Electrophysiologic and retinal penetration studies following intravitreal injection of bevacizumab (Avastin). Retina 2006; 26:262-9.

[27] 24. Rosenfeld PJ, Schwartz SD, Blumenkranz MS, et al. Maximum tolerated dose of a humanized anti-vascular endothelial growth factor antibody fragment for treating neovascular age-related macular degeneration. Ophthalmology 2005;112: 1048–53.

[28] 25. Rosenfeld PJ, Moshfeghi AA, Puliafito CA. Optical coherence tomography findings after an intravitreal injection of bevacizumab (Avastin) for neovascular age-related macular degeneration. Ophthalmic Surg Lasers Imaging 2005;36:331–5.

[29] 26. Avery RL, Pieramici DJ, Rabena MD, et al. Intravitreal bevacizumab (Avastin) for neovascular age-related macular degeneration. Ophthalmology 2006;113:363–72.

[30] 27. Bashshur ZF, Bazarbachi A, Schakal A, et al. Intravitreal bevacizumab for the management of choroidal eovascularization in age-related macular degeneration. Am J Ophthalmol 2006;142:1–9.

[31] Q. D. Nguyen, J. Heier, D. Brown et al., "Randomized, doublemasked, active-controlled phase 3 trial of the efficacy and safety of intravitreal VEGF-Trap-Eye in wet AMD: one-year results of the VIEW-1 study," in Proceedings of the Association for Research in Vision and Ophthalmology, no. 3073, Fort Lauderdale, Fla, USA, 2011.

[32] U. Schmidt-Erfurth, V. Chong, B. Kirchhof et al., "Primary results of an international phase III study using intravitreal VEGF Trap-Eye compared to ranibizumab in patients with wet AMD (VIEW2)," in Proceedings of the Association for Research in Vision and Ophthalmology, no. 1650, Fort Lauderdale, Fla, USA, 2011.

[33] Brown DM, Heier JS, Ciulla T, Benz M, Abraham P, Yancopoulos G, Stahl N, Ingerman A, Vitti R, Berliner AJ, Yang K, Nguyen QD; CLEAR-IT 2 Investigators. Primary endpoint results of a phase II study of vascular endothelial growth factor trap-eye in wet age-related macular degeneration. Ophthalmology. 2011 ;118(6):1089-97.

[34] G. A. Lalwani, P. J. Rosenfeld, A. E. Fung et al., "A variable dosing regimen with intravitreal ranibizumab for neovascular age-related macular degeneration: year 2 of the PrONTO study," American Journal of Ophthalmology, vol. 148, no. 1, pp.1–3, 2009.

[35] F. G. Holz,W. Amoaku, J. Donate et al., "Safety and efficacy of a flexible dosing regimen of ranibizumab in neovascular agerelated macular degeneration: the SUSTAIN study," Ophthalmology, vol. 118, no. 4, pp. 663–671, 2011.

[36] Boyer DS, Heier JS, Brown DM, Francom SF, Ianchulev T, Rubio RG. A Phase IIIb study to evaluate the safety of ranibizumab in subjects with neovascular age-related macular degeneration. Ophthalmology. 2009 Sep;116(9):1731-9.

[37] Singer MA, Awh CC, Sadda S, Freeman WR, Antoszyk AN, Wong P, Tuomi L.HORIZON: An Open-Label Extension Trial of Ranibizumab for Choroidal Neovascularization Secondary to Age-Related Macular Degeneration. Ophthalmology. 2012 ;119(6): 1175-83.

[38] Tano Y, Ohji M . ; EXTEND-I Study Group. Long-term efficacy and safety of ranibizumab administered pro re nata in Japanese patients with neovascular age-related macular degeneration in the EXTEND-I study. Acta Ophthalmol. 2011 ;89(3):208-17

[39] M. Engelbert, S. A. Zweifel, and K. B. Freund, ""treat and extend" dosing of intravitreal antivascular endothelial growth factor therapy for type 3 neovascularization/ retinal angiomatous proliferation," Retina, vol. 29, no. 10, pp. 1424–1431, 2009.

[40] H.Oubraham, S. Y. Cohen, S. Samimi et al., "Inject and extend dosing versus dosing as needed: a comparative retrospective study of ranibizumab in exudative age-related macular degeneration," Retina, vol. 31, no. 1, pp. 26–30, 2010.

[41] O. P. Gupta, G. Shienbaum, A. H. Patel, C. Fecarotta, R. S. Kaiser, and C. D. Regillo, "A treat and extend regimen using ranibizumab for neovascular age-related macular degeneration: clinical and economic impact," Ophthalmology, vol. 117, no. 11, pp. 2134–2140, 2010.

[42] A. Tufail, P. J. Patel, C. Egan et al., "Bevacizumab for neovascular age related macular degeneration (ABC Trial): multicenter randomised double masked study," British Medical Journal, vol. 340, no. 7761, Article ID c2459, p. 1398, 2010.

[43] K. C. S. Fong, N. Kirkpatrick, Q. Mohamed, and R. L.Johnston, "Intravitreal bevacizumab (Avastin) for neovascular age-related macular degeneration using a variable frequency regimen in eyes with no previous treatment," Clinical and Experimental Ophthalmology, vol. 36, no. 8, pp. 748–755, 2008.

[44] P. J. Mekjavic, A. Kraut, and M. Urbancic, "Efficacy of 12-month treatment of neovascular age-related macular degeneration with intravitreal bevacizumab based on individually determined injection strategies after three consecutive monthly injections," Acta Ophthalmologica, vol. 89, no. 7, pp. 647–653, 2009.

[45] S. T. Luu, T. Gray, S. K. Warrier et al., "Retrospective study of an as required dosing regimen of intravitreal bevacizumab in neovascular age-related macular degeneration in an Australian population," Clinical and Experimental Ophthalmology, vol. 38, no. 7, pp. 659–663, 2010.

[46] J. F. Arevalo, J. G. Snchez, L. Wu et al., "Intravitreal bevacizumab for subfoveal choroidal neovascularization in age related macular degeneration at twenty-four months: the panamerican collaborative retina study," Ophthalmology, vol. 117, no. 10, pp. 1974–1981, 2010.

[47] Z. F. Bashshur, Z. A. Haddad, A. R. Schakal, R. F. Jaafar, A. Saad, and B. N. Noureddin, "Intravitreal bevacizumab for treatment of neovascular age-related macular degeneration: the second year of a prospective study," American Journal of Ophthalmology, vol. 148, no. 1, pp. 59–65, 2009.

[48] "Treat-and-extend therapy a popular, cost-effective approach to treating neovascular AMD," PCONSuperSite, 2011.

[49] D. F. Martin, M. G. Maguire, G. -S. Ying, J. E. Grunwald, S. L. Fine, and G. J. Jaffe, "Ranibizumab and bevacizumab for neovascular age-related macular degeneration," New England Journal of Medicine, vol. 364, no. 20, pp. 1897–1908, 2011.

[50] P. J. Rosenfeld, "Bevacizumab versus ranibizumab—the verdict," New England Journal of Medicine, vol. 364, no. 20, pp. 1966–1967, 2011.

[51] Comparison of Age-related Macular Degeneration Treatments Trials (CATT) Research Group, Martin DF, Maguire MG, Fine SL, Ying GS, Jaffe GJ, Grunwald JE, Toth C, Redford M, Ferris FL 3rd. Ranibizumab and Bevacizumab for Treatment of Neovascular Age-related Macular Degeneration: Two-Year Results. Ophthalmology. 2012 Jul;119(7):1388-98.

[52] The IVAN Study Investigators(□) Writing Committee:, Chakravarthy U, Harding SP, Rogers CA, Downes SM, Lotery AJ, Wordsworth S, Reeves BC Ranibizumabversus-Bevacizumab to TreatNeovascularAge-related Macular Degeneration: One-Year Findings from the IVAN Randomized Trial.Ophthalmology. 2012 May 10. [Epub ahead of print]

[53] VIBERA Study. www.clinicaltrials.gov. NCT00559715.

[54] EQUAL studyhttp://www.trialregister.nl/trialreg/admin/rctview.asp?TC=1331

[55] Manta Study. www.clinicaltrials.gov. NCT00710229.

[56] J. S. Slakter, "What to do when anti-VEGF therapy fails," Retinal Physician, 2010.

[57] A. Y. Lee, A. K. Raya, S. M. Kymes, A. Shiels, andM. A. Brantley, "Pharmacogenetics of complement factor H (Y402H) and treatment of exudative age-related macular degeneration with ranibizumab," British Journal of Ophthalmology, vol. 93, no. 5, pp. 610–613, 2009.

[58] M. A. Brantley, A. M. Fang, J. M. King, A. Tewari, S. M. Kymes, and A. Shiels, "Association of complement factor H and LOC387715 genotypes with response of exudative age related macular degeneration to intravitreal bevacizumab,"Ophthalmology, vol. 114, no. 12, pp. 2168–2173, 2007.

[59] Larsen M, Schmidt-Erfurth U, Lanzetta P, Wolf S, Simader C, Tokaji E, Pilz S, Weisberger A; MONT BLANC Study Group. Verteporfin plus ranibizumab for choroidal neovascularization in age-related macular degeneration: twelve-month MONT BLANC study results. Ophthalmology. 2012 May;119(5):992-1000

[60] Kaiser PK, Boyer DS, Cruess AF, Slakter JS, Pilz S, Weisberger A; DENALI Study Group. Verteporfin plus ranibizumab for choroidal neovascularization in age-related macular degeneration: twelve-month results of the DENALI study. Ophthalmology. 2012 May;119(5):1001-10

[61] Piermarocchi S, Sartore M, Lo Giudice G, Maritan V, Midena E, and Segato T. Combination of photodynamic therapy and intraocular triamcinolone for exudative age-related macular degeneration and long-term chorioretinal macular atrophy. Archives of Ophthalmology 2008;126(10): 1367–1374.

[62] Iwama D, Otani A, Sasahara M, Yodoi Y, Gotoh N, Tamura H, Tsujikawa A, and Yoshimura N. Photodynamic therapy combined with low-dose intravitreal triamcinolone acetonide for age-related macular degeneration refractory to photodynamic therapy alone. British Journal of Ophthalmology 2008;92(10): 1352–1356.

[63] Blaha GR, Wertz IFD, and Marx JL. Profound choroidal hypoperfusion after combined photodynamic therapy and intravitreal triamcinolone acetonide. Ophthalmic Surgery Lasers and Imaging 2008;39(1): 6–11.

[64] Rodrigues EB, Grumann A, Jr., Penha FM, et al. Effect of needle type and injection technique on pain level and vitreal reflux in intravitreal injection. Journal of Ocular Pharmacology and Therapeutics. 2011;27:197–203.

[65] Ta CN. Minimizing the risk of endophthalmitis following intravitreous injections. Retina 2004;24:699 –705.

[66] Lauer G, Sollberg S, Cole M, et al. Expression and proteolysis of vascular endothelial growth factor is increased in chronic wounds. J Invest Dermatol 2000;115:12– 8.

[67] Carmeliet P, Ng YS, Nuyens D, et al. Impaired myocardial angiogenesis and ischemic cardiomyopathy in mice lacking the vascular endothelial growth factor isoforms VEGF164 and VEGF188. Nat Med 1999;5:495–502.

[68] Rosamond W, Flegal K, Friday G, et al. Heart disease and stroke statistics—2007 update: a report from the American Heart Association Statistics Committee and Stroke Statistics Subcommittee. Circulation 2007;115:e69 –171.

[69] S. Barik, "Development of gene-specific double-stranded RNA drugs," Annals of Medicine, vol. 36, no. 7, pp. 540–551, 2004.

[70] M. J. Tolentino, A. J. Brucker, J. Fosnot et al., "Intravitreal injection of vascular endothelial growth factor small interfering RNA inhibits growth and leakage in a nonhuman primate, laser-induced model of choroidal neovascularization," Retina, vol. 24, no. 1, pp. 132–138, 2004.

[71] M. J. Tolentino, A. J. Brucker, J. Y. Fosnot et al., "Intravitreal injection of vascular endothelial growth factor small interfering RNA inhibits growth and leakage in the nonhuman primate, laser-induced model of choroidal neovascularization," Retina, vol. 24, no. 4, p. 660, 2004.

[72] A. O. Garba and S. A. Mousa, "Bevasiranib for the treatment of wet age-related macular degeneration," Journal of Ophthalmology and Eye Diseases, vol. 2, pp. 75–83, 2010.

[73] J. Perkel, "RNAi therapeutics: a two-year update," Science, vol. 326, pp. 454–456, 2009.

[74] Kaiser PK: Antivascular endothelial growth factor agents and their development: therapeutic implications in ocular diseases. Am J Ophthalmol 2006;142:660–668.

[75] Safety and Efficacy of Oral PTK787 in Patients with Subfoveal Choroidal Neovascularization Secondary to Age-Related Macular Degeneration (AMD) (ADVANCE). http://www.clinicaltrials.gov/ct2/show/NCT00138632?order=1 (accessed October 02, 2012).

[76] Sonpavde G, Hutson TE, Sternberg CN: Pazopanib, a potent orally administered small-molecule multitargeted tyrosine kinase inhibitor for renal cell carcinoma. Expert Opin Investig Drugs 2008;17:253–261.

[77] A Study to Evaluate the Pharmacodynamics, Safety, and Pharmacokinetics of Pazopanib Drops in Adult Subjects with Neovascular AMD. http://www.clinicaltrials.gov/ct2/show/ NCT00612456?order=1 (accessed October 02, 2012).

[78] Wigginton JM, Gruys E, Geiselhart L, Subleski J, Komschlies KL, Park JW, Wiltrout TA, Nagashima K, Back TC, Wiltrout RH: IFN-gamma and Fas/FasL are required for the antitumor and antiangiogenic effects of IL-12/pulse IL-2 therapy. J Clin Invest 2001;108:51–62.

[79] Mochimaru H, Nagai N, Hasegawa G, Kudo-Saito C, Yaguchi T, Usui Y, et al: Suppression of choroidal neovascularization by dendritic cell vaccination targeting VEGFR2. Invest Ophthalmol Vis Sci 2007;48:4795–4801.

[80] Anti-VEGFR Vaccine Therapy in Treating Patients with Neovascular Maculopathy. http://www.clinicaltrials.gov/ct2/show/NCT00791570?order=1 (accessed October 02, 2012).

[81] Nozaki M, Raisler BJ, Sakuri E, Baffi JZ, Ambati BK, Ambati J: Drusen complement components C3. Proc Natl Acad Sci USA 2006;103:2328–2333.

[82] AMD Patients Treated with POT-4 Demonstrate No Adverse Toxic Effects during Phase I Clinical Trial. http://www.medicalnewstoday.com/articles/128837.php (accessed October 02, 2012).

[83] ARC1905 (ANTI-C5 APTAMER) Given either in Combination Therapy with Lucentis® 0.5 mg/Eye in Subjects with Neovascular Age-Related Macular Degeneration. http://www.clinicaltrials.gov/ct2/show/ NCT00709527?order=1 (accessed October 02, 2012).

[84] Treating Wet Form of AMD – Othera Eye Drop Data Shows Synergistic Effect with Lucentis and Avastin. http://www.medicalnewstoday.com/articles/63892.php (accessed October 02, 2012).

[85] OT-551 Antioxidant Eye Drops to Treat Geographic Atrophy in Age-Related Macular Degeneration. http://clinicaltrials.gov/ct2/show/NCT00306488 (accessed October 02, 2012).

[86] Mori K, Gehlbach P, Ando A, McVey D, Wei L, Campochiaro PA: Regression of ocular neovascularization in response to increased expression of pigment epithelium-derived factor. Invest Ophthalmol Vis Sci 2002;43:2428–2434.\

[87] Campochiaro PA, Nguyen QD, Shah SM, Klein ML, Holz E, Frank RN, et al: Adenoviral vector-delivered pigment epithelium-derived factor for neovascular age-related macular degeneration: results of a phase I clinical trial. Hum Gene Ther 2006;17:167–176